PEACEFUL PREGNANCY MEDITATIONS

*A Diary
For Expectant Mothers*

By Lisa Steele George, M.A.

Health Communications, Inc.
Deerfield Beach, Florida

©1993 Lisa Steele George
ISBN 1-55874-263-8

All rights reserved. Printed in the United States of America. No part of this publication may be reproduced, stored in a retrieval system or transmitted in any form or by any means, electronic, mechanical, photocopying, recording or otherwise without the written permission of the publisher.

Publisher: Health Communications, Inc.
          3201 S.W. 15th Street
          Deerfield Beach, Florida 33442-8190

Cover design by Andrea Perrine

Dedications

To

To my dad, Robert John, whose continued spiritual strength and trust has been a gift to me for I have learned the importance of staying close to God and that every day is truly a gift.

To

To Joseph A. Sommer, S.J., who taught so many the true meaning of affirmation, humor and faith.

To

To Dalton Robert, without whose precious presence this work would not exist. Thank you for adding such sweetness to our lives.

Acknowledgments

Loving thanks to my husband David who supported me throughout the creation of this book, from the visionary stage to the final manuscript. Not only did he constantly give feedback on my ideas, but he also offered useful advice from a male/father/husband viewpoint. His tremendous commitment and dedication in our lives are always a source of strength and saving grace.

I am especially grateful to my parents for always believing in my visions and dreams. Their generosity, love and care have given me much of the strength I need for being a parent.

A special thank you to Ellie Mitchell Caldwell who fine-tuned this book with her editing skills.

To Barbara Nichols for believing in this work and Gail Chernoff for her support and direction.

Grateful thoughts to my doctor, Andrew Check, for his constant sharing of information, comforting words and expertise throughout my pregnancy, and to Linda Simler, his office manager, for the many kind words of encouragement and friendly atmosphere she so easily creates.

Introduction

When I became pregnant with Dalton, I knew there would be anxious times. I felt that the more I knew about this adventure, the less anxious I would feel. So I did what many expectant mothers do. I read everything I could find about the physical and medical aspects of being pregnant. I talked with other expectant mothers about their experiences and inundated my doctor and my older sister Cindy with questions. But something was still missing.

By the end of my second trimester I realized that I had found neither daily emotional support nor an outlet for the myriad feelings, moods and shifting attitudes that went along with being pregnant. With this revelation came the birth of this book. I wrote meditations every day on what I felt, feared or was experiencing. When I stayed in touch with my fears and feelings, they were less likely to catch me off guard. And when I considered the role of my benevolent Higher Power during my pregnancy, a sense of spirituality developed which left me more at peace and seemed to have a calming effect.

I hope you write your own feelings, thoughts or affirmations each day.

These meditations and journal keepsakes are my gifts to you in hopes of helping you to have a *Peaceful Pregnancy*, too.

Lisa Steele George

Contents

1. First Trimester 1
2. Second Trimester 97
3. Third Trimester 193
4. Overdue Addendum 277

First Trimester

Beginnings

Day 1

When does pregnancy really begin? At conception? Years ago when we started yearning for a family of our own? Yesterday when our home pregnancy test turned positive? For each mother-to-be, it is different. But no matter where we define our beginning, we know it is truly that: a new beginning.

Some of us may have taken a long time to get here. Mornings of taking our temperature and depression over recurring periods. Nights of "planned" lovemaking and possibly visits to fertility specialists. Congratulations to us for sticking to our hopes and dreams!

Today is a new beginning.
I look toward the fresh beginning of a new life.

Date / /

Today I Feel _____

Creation

Day 2

Someone once said everything is created twice: first time in our minds and then in reality. Before we were pregnant, we may not have understood the meaning behind this statement. But now that we carry life within us, every day we think about what our baby will look like, how we will be as parents and even what the baby's room will look like. We are creating ideas of things that are not here yet, but will be. Parenthood, for us, is an experience that we now see is created twice.

Remembering my thoughts are predecessors of a new creation helps me to realize the importance of positive imaging.

Date / /

Today I Feel _____

_____

_____

_____

Secrets

Day 3

Being pregnant can be the best kept secret ever! Since every woman is really the only one who knows her menstrual cycle, being able to keep this secret is easy, at least for a while. There may be many reasons why we would want to: fear of an early miscarriage, uncertainty about having a child, or others' possible anger, blame or lack of care. Or our pregnancy may seem too personal to share at this point. Whatever the reason, it is important that we don't lie to ourselves. We need to assess honestly *why* we are keeping this secret. Is it healthy? For power or control? Fear?

Why haven't I shared my news?
Do I lack trust in my friends or even my Higher Power?

Date / /

Today I Feel _____

_____
_____
_____

Worry

Day 4

We may discover that we have been pregnant for quite a few weeks without knowing it. Then we start to worry about what we have been doing: drinking coffee, taking over-the-counter drugs or smoking cigarettes. Worry is normal and quite often present during pregnancy. Let's recognize it now and do what we can to improve our habits. We should not let worry consume us during this happy time. As long as we are now getting medical attention and taking care of ourselves, it has never been safer to have a baby.

*As I focus on my early pregnancy,
I let go of the past and concentrate on
good care in the present.*

Date / /

Today I Feel

Conception

Day 5

Why do we bother trying to figure out exactly when conception occurred? Was it the night of our friend's party? Last Sunday morning? That ski trip? When will our questioning stop? And will we ever really know?

We want to feel secure that the circumstances were "right." We fear that conception might have happened at the wrong time. Were we drinking? Was our mate? Were we feeling healthy? Happy?

We are seeing ourselves as completely responsible for the condition of conception and the early development of our baby. Who are we kidding? Do we really think we are anything but God's assistants?

I let go of my need to control and see my life held in the hands of a loving God.

Date / /

Today I Feel _____

False Alarms

Day 6

Imagination, stress, nerves, call it what we may, but we have missed another period. Another home pregnancy test has proved positive. Are we really pregnant after all this waiting or is this another false alarm? Having faced so much failure before, we are afraid of further disappointment.

What we need to do is set aside our fears and make an appointment with the doctor again, just to be sure. We want the best start for our baby. We need to know if we are pregnant so we can start vitamins and planning.

What do I really have to lose by going to the doctor? Not much compared to what I could potentially be gaining.

Date / /

Today I Feel _____

Purpose

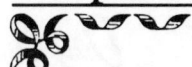

Day 7

Prior to our pregnancy we had goals set: a job, social events or hobbies. But now, our lives have taken on a new purpose. Our pregnancy deepens the meaning of our everyday existence. It creates an unselfish heart within us and brings the gift of unconditional love.

Now, our most important goal is a healthy and safe pregnancy. We need to work to stay on the path of a healthy lifestyle. We can no longer be satisfied for doing things "just for ourselves." Inappropriate behaviors, such as drinking or smoking, rob us of a peaceful heart and steer us away from fulfilling our main purpose at this time in our lives.

Everything else that I do must come second now because this baby only has one chance of developing properly.

Date   /   /

Today I Feel _____

_____

_____

_____

Power

Day 8

We can choose to have a positive attitude toward our pregnancy with the power of our own inner strength. We do not have to listen to those around us. If other pregnant friends are not taking care of themselves, we can express concern, but we need to concentrate on our own care. We can make the effort to change ourselves, but we don't need to use our precious energy trying to control others. If we just relax and let things unfold, we will enjoy our pregnancy much more than trying to superimpose our will on everyone else.

*The more I concentrate on myself now,
the more personal power I have
and the happier I am.*

Date / /

Today I Feel

Medical Information

Day 9

As we start our prenatal care, we may need to disclose medical history that is difficult to talk about. Perhaps we have high blood pressure from not taking care of ourselves, a previous abortion, problems from sexual contacts or even past abuse that makes physical contact painful. Being honest with our doctor is a responsible act and can help avoid risks to our unborn child. Whatever our past, we must remind ourselves that it's over and beyond our control. Now we need to concentrate on taking care of ourselves and getting the help we need for a healthy pregnancy.

*I take responsibility for my health and
do what I can to improve it.*

Date / /

Today I Feel _____

_____

_____

_____

Say No

Day 10

Our baby cannot say no to potentially harmful substances, but we can. If we have improved our mental and physical health for this pregnancy, we can congratulate ourselves. Healthy attitudes and behaviors are the best way to help our pregnancy and have a healthy baby. Many studies have shown the powerful effects of harmful substances on the developing fetus. Although most days we feel very strong, happy and content, other days the anxieties may seem overpowering and a drink or a chocolate binge may seem appealing. But we know deep within us that a healthy lifestyle is important for the life we carry within.

I continue to say no to unhealthy behaviors in my life, for both my benefit and my baby's.

Date   /   /

Today I Feel _____

Greater Power

Day 11

What role does God play in our lives? Are we open to the idea of a Higher Power guiding us throughout our pregnancy?

If we give the spiritual side a chance to grow during this pregnancy, we will experience greater peace and healing. A Power greater than us will carry a lot of our worries and burdens. The more we learn to depend on this Power, the more peacefully connected we feel with ourselves and our families. Our faith helps us let go and let God manage our lives.

Spirituality plays a major role in keeping me sane during my pregnancy and gives me hope and a needed sense of peace.

Date / /

Today I Feel _____

Doubters

Day 12

Friends and family may have some difficulty accepting our pregnancy. They may have questions, concerns, and even worry. We do not have to let them affect us and our moods. We need to surround ourselves with supportive people who bolster our confidence and lend a helping hand. But what can we do with the "doubters"? We need to communicate that we do not appreciate their comments, ignore or avoid them, prepare answers ahead of time so that we are not caught off guard or simply change the subject outright. All in all, we need to take control to eliminate or decrease the "doubters" in our lives.

It is important that I feel good about my decisions, surrounding myself with supporters, not "doubters."

Date / /

Today I Feel

Announcement

Day 13

Feeling special is something we don't experience enough in our lives. Now that we are pregnant, we may be feeling this natural high repeat itself every time we announce the news to another person. We will never forget the day or place when we discovered our pregnancy. Why not take the extra effort to make the announcement special to others?

Are we near Mother's Day? What better day to announce it to our mothers? Do our kids associate turkey dinner with special occasions? We can announce it to them after a special dinner together. Do we have a special place we take walks with our husbands? Why not walk there on a beautiful night and share the wonderful news?

I announce my pregnancy with the attention it deserves and create special memories of this moment.

Date / /

Today I Feel _____

_____

_____

_____

Fear

Day 14

Have we really been frightened since we found out we're pregnant? Have we not confided in anyone because we are still in shock? And most importantly, have we not sought medical attention because we are still uncomfortable with our situation?

Finding ourselves pregnant is a very emotional experience, particularly if it is unplanned, but delaying medical care increases the chances of physical complications for us and the fetus. The first trimester is the most important for developing a healthy baby and we need to begin medical care, taking vitamins and iron and eating well.

Even if I am unsure of my situation, it is important to take good care of myself now.

Date / /

Today I Feel _____

_____

_____

_____

Choice

Day 15

While we may not control the reality of our pregnancy, we can choose how to respond to it. At first, this may seem difficult, especially if it is unplanned. But through the help of our Higher Power, we can choose how to respond to our condition in the best way for us.

Going somewhere to be alone gives us the chance to accept our condition both emotionally and spiritually. We may need a conversation with God or with ourselves or some quiet time just to sit or to write in a journal. By doing this, we'll be able to feel composed, more in charge of our attitudes.

*By choosing my attitudes consciously,
I am responsible to myself and my pregnancy.*

Date / /

Today I Feel _____

_____

_____

_____

Gifts

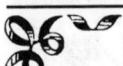

Day 16

A list of all the gifts in our lives would be never-ending, with our pregnancy at the very top. Each event and person is a precious gift with an important purpose. This perspective becomes even more apparent after our baby is born, as we see a new life unfold.

Many good things are in our lives right now: reflections of what our world offers and what our baby will be a part of. A safe and secure home, filled with love, is a wonderful first gift to share with our baby.

Today it is easy to get drawn into the complex material world dominated by commodities. But our spirit recognizes the simple and small gifts of our lives.

The more I recognize that everything in my life is a gift, the more peaceful I am.

Date   /   /

Today I Feel _____

Leadership

Day 17

Do we consider our pregnancy an opportunity to be a leader? Leadership is so often associated with the work environment that we forget its role in our personal lives. Being pregnant is a good chance to practice leadership skills to create the environment we need for a healthy pregnancy.

Being a leader does not mean giving orders or expecting others to wait on us. Complaining all the time or not taking care of ourselves is not leading or gaining the support of others. Leadership during pregnancy is the ability to motivate my family and friends so they will help me reach my goal of having a healthy pregnancy and birth.

*I can be a leader role model
throughout my pregnancy and motivate
others to help out.*

Date   /   /

Today I Feel _____

_____

_____

Hope

Day 18

Now that we are pregnant, we may find ourselves reflecting a lot on our life. It becomes easy to think of our shortcomings. Maybe we should have worked on developing better relationships, obtaining financial security or purchasing a secure home. Perhaps we feel we should have a better job or more education. All of these thoughts may create a sense of anger about our present situation. Instead of dwelling on this emotion, what about redirecting ourselves toward hope? Hope for an improved life!

With my baby comes a new sense of hope, hope for a better tomorrow full of many new beginnings.

Date / /

Today I Feel _____

Siblings

Day 19

As second-time expectant mothers we may worry we won't love a second child as much as we did our first. We adored our first babies and have such a deep love for them. We fear that this won't be duplicated with another child. Our next baby may not seem as cute, fun, sweet, loving or healthy.

Our fears are misplaced. We will have the same bonding with our new baby and we *do* have the ability to love both simultaneously.

All babies have their own personalities, physical features and developmental stages. We can trust that we will instinctively be able to nurture our newest little miracle.

I trust that I will have the inner resources
to love my second child and look forward to seeing
this child's beauty unfold before me.

Date / /

Today I Feel _____

_____

_____

_____

Intentions

Day 20

What intentions do we have with this pregnancy? Did we get pregnant to bring us closer to our partner? To have our partner make a commitment? Or were we ready to begin a family together? Understanding our motives helps us cope with our pregnancy. But no matter what the intention, we have a precious life developing within us and we need to make sure our choices are now on the right track. Through positive planning, we establish healthy habits that create a healthy pregnancy and birth. With the right motives we gain confidence in our ability to be positive expectant parents.

Each day I give my best effort to ensure the health of myself and my unborn child.

Date / /

Today I Feel _____

_____

_____

_____

Lifestyle

Day 21

Having spiritual and emotional well-being is only part of feeling whole, balanced and healthy. We need to extend our nurturing to ourselves to facilitate a healthy pregnancy.

So many times we try to do what our minds tell us, like staying up too late or finishing errands at the mall when our back hurts. Taking the time to listen to our bodies, we can avoid later problems.

In addition, we may find ourselves leaning toward poor nutritional habits. We need to remind ourselves gently that these offenders will only contribute to our emotional imbalance and subsequent weight problems.

Every day I choose the healthiest lifestyle possible as I build a good relationship between body and mind.

Date / /

Today I Feel _____

Relationship

Day 22

Having a baby means that our marriage will never be the same. Any long-term relationship endures many changes over the years due to growth and life changes. Just like any other major change in our relationship, such as buying a house or getting a new job, pregnancy will have a great impact.

Pregnancy can be viewed, though, as one of the natural developmental stages of our married life. Instead of labeling it a "major change," we can see it as a passage from one stage to the next. Our relationship with our spouse is growing, and where there is growth, there is bound to be change.

Being pregnant means change is beckoning at my door. May I greet it eagerly!

Date / /

Today I Feel _____

Guarded Joy

Day 23

Miscarriage may be on our minds throughout this first trimester, the time when we are most at risk. Especially if we had a miscarriage before, we may feel a guarded joy about being pregnant.

Now it is important that we develop healthy habits and give special attention to our bodies. We need to be on the lookout for warning signals. Catching something early may prevent problems. We improve our chances of a healthy pregnancy by taking care of ourselves and getting the medical attention we need. This mindset at the beginning builds a good foundation for the next forty weeks.

I stay aware of my body during pregnancy and give myself the care I need.

Date / /

Today I Feel _____

Acceptance

Day 24

Accepting the reality of this pregnancy may be difficult, particularly if it seems like the "wrong time." It may be the result of a lack of planning. Feeling our anger is a healthy step toward accepting our situation.

One way to cope may be sharing with a close friend or family member. Or we may just want to sit down, have a good cry and go for a long walk to think things through.

Anger is healthy as long as we acknowledge it and don't bottle it up. Perhaps we can also direct the energy into something constructive, such as shopping, cleaning the house, doing laundry or washing the car.

Feeling my anger is healthy, but now I need to move on and accept this developing miracle.

Date / /

Today I Feel _____

_____

_____

_____

Emotional Vulnerability

Day 25

Being emotionally vulnerable goes with being pregnant, from conception to birth. Never before have we felt so easily stirred and so motivated by feelings, not reason. This means we may need to protect ourselves from some undesirable or injurious feelings.

First, we need to delay making any major decisions until the baby is born and our situation becomes more stable. Second, we need to grant ourselves tremendous patience and avoid anxiety if possible. Finally, we need to depend on those we trust in our lives for guidance and support, especially our Higher Power.

Being aware of my emotional vulnerability is the first step in protecting myself from making wrong decisions and hasty reactions.

Date / /

Today I Feel _____

Alternative Insemination

Day 26

Expectant mothers are usually married and pregnant from an act of love between two people. We, on the other hand, may not fit into this norm. We may have chosen alternative insemination to get pregnant, a very planned, methodical procedure. This unconventional choice may bring extra stress, whether we are married, gay, single or divorced.

We are concerned that the baby will be different or worry about the medical procedures we had to go through. We may even have doubts about the unknown donor. In addition, other people may be critical of our choice, telling us it is unnatural or wrong.

*I have the right to share my life with a baby and
I trust God to guide me in all my choices.*

Date   /   /

Today I Feel _____

_____

_____

_____

Heat

Day 27

If we are one of those people who are chilly most of the time, we may be in for a surprise! During pregnancy, a woman's temperature often rises to provide for the needs of the developing child, a luxury we may well enjoy ourselves.

When most people are wearing turtlenecks and suit jackets around the office, we may feel comfortable in a light blouse or T-shirt. Although this may seem like a benefit in winter climates, beware of arguments over the thermostat!

Whether or not my rise in temperature feels good to me, this is just another example of how God ensures that my body fulfills the needs of my baby.

Date   /   /

Today I Feel _____

Abortion

Day 28

At a time when we are feeling overwhelmed with joy, fleeting memories of a previous abortion may bother us. We thought these memories were gone forever, but remorse and grief may return as our new gift of life reminds us of a previous pregnancy we chose to end. Looking back, we realize we chose abortion as a way to solve a difficult problem, which was a right choice at the time.

In order to let go of the past, we must forgive ourselves for the choices of years ago. We need to be able to put this experience behind us and greet our impending future with happiness in our hearts.

*I work through these emotions about
the past and remind myself how blessed I am
to be given a second chance.*

Date   /   /

Today I Feel _____

Timelessness

Day 29

For the first time in our lives we may be distinctly aware of the passage of time, every minute of it. Before we were pregnant we had our daily routines, interrupted by an occasional vacation or change at work. But now with every passing hour, we know our baby is developing at a phenomenal pace and our body is reacting to these changes. One moment our baby is a combination of cells, but within weeks the heart is pumping and little hands have formed. Every second is precious as our little human being develops.

Once our baby is born, she or he will continue changing and growing. We need to savor every day of our pregnancy, for the passage of time is a phenomenon that we can never govern but only marvel at.

My pregnancy is really a memory being created.

Date   /   /

Today I Feel _____

_____

_____

_____

Feeling Whole

Day 30

For the first time in our lives, we may be feeling "whole." Our desire to be pregnant has been fulfilled and our wish to have a child to share our love and life has come true. The feeling of *deja vous* may overwhelm us at times. Unexpectedly, our growing baby inside of us does not feel like a stranger at all! Instead, we feel like we have already known him or her our whole life. It is almost as if they have been a part of us and our bigger plan all along.

While I am pregnant, feeling that I have always known my baby is a special, intimate experience that blesses me. What a lovely time in my life!

Date / /

Today I Feel _____

Extremes

Day 31

Everything during our pregnancy may seem extreme, which is quite natural and commonplace. We are either very happy or very sad, crying hysterically or laughing uproariously, exhausted or energized, loving or unapproachable.

During the second trimester, we will feel more in tune with our bodily changes. Most women claim that this time is the most peaceful as they feel a more natural rhythm and flow within themselves. These feelings lead us to become more confident for our last trimester and revitalize us for the labor and birth.

I will not be frightened by emotional extremes. I know I will soon be liberated from this phase of pregnancy.

Date / /

Today I Feel _____
_____
_____
_____

Warnings

Day 32

No one knows our bodies like we do. We know when we are feeling weak, need rest or are in great shape. During pregnancy, we work hard every day to keep ourselves healthy. But unexpected problems may occur when we need to trust our instincts, take responsibility and contact our medical advisors. At this time we don't want to depend upon others to tell us what to do. We ourselves know when our bodies signal a change that we need to notice. This way we learn to trust our inner guidance, so important when we become parents.

I educate myself on warning signs and do not depend on friends for peace of mind.

Date / /

Today I Feel _____

_____

_____

_____

Friends

Day 33

As happy as we are, we may find it difficult to tell our closest friend if she has been trying to get pregnant for years. We know that we must tell her first, before our other friends find out. But how can we tell her something that we know will bring her pain?

There is only one approach: honesty. We need to find the right place and time to share the news. She needs to know we are sensitive to her feelings and we need to be prepared for a myriad of responses. Hopefully our friendship will be able to overcome this potential barrier.

*I now surround myself with supportive people and
I hope my friend chooses to be one of them.*

Date   /   /

Today I Feel _____

Unreal

Day 34

Being pregnant, like other experiences in our lives, may seem a little unreal. We can't feel the growing baby inside us yet. We do have many symptoms and the tests came out positive, but we may still be telling ourselves that it is just PMS, the flu or being overtired. We ask ourselves, "Am I really pregnant?"

We must remind ourselves to be patient and take one day at a time. Live each moment, hour and event. Days will pass so swiftly that before we know it, we will be in our third trimester wondering where all the time went!

I practice patience and enjoy the sequence of events as my pregnancy unfolds. Each day brings newness. Each trimester brings added love.

Date / /

Today I Feel _____

_____

_____

_____

Praise

Day 35

Do we thank our husbands as they place the last strip of wallpaper in the baby's room? Or do we take their contributions for granted? Why are we so quick to criticize, often in detail, yet not quick to show appreciation?

Most likely there are many ways our spouses are helping during our pregnancy. Since they are half of this parenting team, it is vital we acknowledge their participation. The more we express our appreciation, the more they will want to support us.

When those I love praise me, I feel great,
so I will try to reciprocate and show appreciation for them.

Date / /

Today I Feel _____

Thanks

Day 36

One goal for our pregnancy can be thanking God each day for continued good health. Keeping ourselves and our baby healthy requires our care and also a trust in our Higher Power. Hopefully we will have good health throughout the nine months. If not, we can turn to the knowledge of our doctor and the power of spiritual guidance. If there is something we need to do to stay healthy, we should realize its importance and point ourselves in the right direction immediately.

I thank God daily and do what I need to do to keep as healthy as possible.

Date / /

Today I Feel

Marriage

Day 37

We may be asking ourselves lately if pregnancy is a good reason to get married. Years ago, the answer would have been a quick "yes." At that time women endured any circumstance to provide their child with a father and financial security.

The pressure to marry still exists to some extent. If we love the father we may decide to get married. But this may not be right, especially if we've only known him a short time. Marriage adds responsibility and commitment that we may not be ready for.

We need to carefully analyze the reasons for considering marriage.

*One key question I can ask myself is,
"Would I marry this person anyway?"*

Date / /

Today I Feel _____

Rugged Strength

Day 38

Where do we get our strength? From our spouse? A friend? Besides these sources of support, we need to discover our inner resources. By depending on ourselves and our Higher Power we gain confidence to create a peaceful pregnancy.

When we are feeling alone and confused, we can search into our souls for rugged strength from our Higher Power. There we find not only the strength to flourish, but also the ability to bear whatever our pregnancy brings. God never fails to hear our call for help or send whatever support we need.

Others in my life provide support,
but the best source is within, through
contact with my Higher Power.

Date / /

Today I Feel _____

Guilt

Day 39

Announcing our pregnancy, we sit back and watch how people react. Unfortunately, such happy news may disturb some people. Our parents may dislike the idea that they are old enough to be grandparents. A sister may feel judgmental if we are not married. Or our partner may be upset because we do not yet have financial security.

But we are the ones carrying this baby and we want this to be a new beginning. Before we announce our pregnancy, we need to think this through so we are not made to feel uncomfortable by others.

If others are upset about my pregnancy, I will remind myself that they're reacting to how the situation affects them and it's really their problem, not mine.

Date / /

Today I Feel _____

Infertility

Day 40

If we have experienced years of infertility and were told we would never have children, our pregnancy is truly an occasion to celebrate! The question may be, though, do we still want children? We may actually have become quite comfortable with our childless lifestyle. We enjoy coming and going as we please, sleeping through the night and having minimum responsibilities. How will we manage to change now?

We need to remember that we do not have to change overnight. Nature has been generous, giving us nine months to adjust.

I have faith that in due time I will become comfortable with the gift of my pregnancy and look forward to the child coming into our lives.

Date / /

Today I Feel _____

_____

_____

_____

Resentment

Day 41

Pregnancy can be an unpleasant time, with various physical and emotional problems. We are disappointed at not having the "perfect pregnancy" we dreamed of. The reality may be difficult, especially if we start to feel out of control.

We also may begin to feel resentment toward the baby, blaming it for our difficulties. Deep down we know our baby is innocent and we should not blame it. Such attitudes are often characteristic of pregnancy itself, not just ours alone. Negative emotions are a normal reaction to a physical experience that is turning our lives upside down.

I will try to adjust better to this pregnancy and not let resentment overwhelm me.

Date / /

Today I Feel

Sharing News

Day 42

Suspense builds as we wait by the phone for news on the result of a pregnancy test. Or we are taken by surprise when the doctor says, "By the way, you're pregnant." Tears well up as we find out we're seven weeks along. As prepared as we thought we were, we still feel shocked but we also feel joy and fear. We leave the office and drive home carrying this awesome news with us.

We may wait to share the news with others, excitedly telling only our partner. He, too, now knows this wonderful secret. It is a time to cherish as we become used to the change in our lives.

*Telling others is my decision when both
my partner and I are ready.*

Date / /

Today I Feel _____

In Tune

Day 43

At no other time in our lives have we ever been so in tune with our bodies and aware of every feature and part. A day does not pass without our looking into a mirror for changes and growth in our hair, skin or nails. We analyze our abdomens, legs and ankles and realize that God is in full control of this process. We feel more in tune with Mother Nature and her gifts to the world: the gentle animals and their offspring, fresh, new greenery and the warm morning sunlight. Mother Nature is flourishing everywhere, just as she should be.

Pregnancy has granted me a new sense of appreciation for my precious, beautiful body and the wonderful gifts of Mother Nature.

Date / /

Today I Feel

Great Days

Day 44

During this time in our lives when so much is happening, it is easy to wake up in the morning feeling anxious. If we find this happening, we must realize that we have the power to choose what kind of day we will have. Each day is a new beginning. The weather, our nausea, our circumstances or other people do not cause our whole day to be a downer. We do.

Each night before we go to bed, we can reflect on our day. What did we like? What did we dislike? How will we do things differently in the future and how will we manage our attitudes differently? We also can reflect on the good things in our day. Then we can make our next day's plans.

I have the power to make this a great day!

Date / /

Today I Feel _____

Demystify

Day 45

One goal throughout these nine months should be to demystify childbirth. This will lead us to feel stronger and more confident about the experience ahead. To accomplish this, we need to ask others for help. We need to experience the power gained by learning from them. Our doctor, coworkers, family and friends can all be sources of help and strength. From them, we learn about ourselves, pregnancy and childbirth. Then we understand better the experience of childbirth so we can make it a more peaceful transition.

I learn about this stage in my life by depending on others, especially the greatest source, my Higher Power.

Date / /

Today I Feel _____

_____

_____

_____

Persistence

Day 46

There will be times during our pregnancy when we wish we could walk away, not just from being pregnant but from our jobs, family, home, doctor and all our responsibilities. We must remember, though, that we will profit from persistence and determination. Even if our original enthusiasm is waning, we will be strengthened if we do not abandon our efforts. As with other endeavors, we are building confidence, strength and character. And, of course, we will also present a beautiful baby to the world and create ourselves as a new mother!

*I drive on and trust that the road
will lead me where I need to go.*

Date / /

Today I Feel

Overwhelmed

Day 47

This is only the beginning and already there are so many things to do. We had been feeling comfortable about our lives and our routines. Now, all of a sudden, there are doctor's appointments, medical tests, childbirth classes and the list is growing. Some days we may feel like giving up. If we need a break, let's just give it to ourselves. Take a day just to remember the minimum and not discuss pregnancy with anyone. We have to try not to overdose now on pregnancy because we have a long route yet to travel.

I will remind myself to take one day at a time and let my Higher Power guide me.

Date / /

Today I Feel _____

Disappointment

Day 48

Not one of us will go through pregnancy (or life) without some disappointment. We intend to meet each day with eager expectation, but unplanned events occur that may upset us. We may be depending on our spouse and he simply isn't there. We may need emotional support from our physician and all we get is criticism. We must remember that none of this is our fault. Our efforts may go unrewarded and expectations may be unfulfilled for reasons we cannot explain. We need to put these experiences behind us and go forward, moving on to a new tomorrow.

I deal with disappointment without letting it consume me.

Date / /

Today I Feel _____

Stress

Day 49

All of us have times when we think negative thoughts about our condition. Some days we wish we were not pregnant or had time to reconsider. We may wonder what is wrong with us for thinking these terrible things. Guilt sets in and we begin to feel out of control. Then worry starts up. What an unrewarding, vicious circle. At this point we may wonder if this mindset will affect our baby. Although thoughts cannot damage our baby, stress can. If negative thinking is occurring because of stress in our lives, we need to recognize this, tell our doctor and give it the attention it deserves.

If I find myself having negative thoughts,
I will find ways to reduce stress in my life.

Date   /   /

Today I Feel _____

_____

_____

_____

Decision-Making

Day 50

Every day we are faced with numerous decisions, some routine, others serious. We have recently made one of the most important: to have a child. We know that this will have a profound effect on our life ahead.

This is only the beginning of many decisions we will make over the coming months. With every new day there are new choices. Fortunately we don't have to make them on our own. We can seek advice from family, friends and our medical advisors. More importantly, we can seek guidance from our Higher Power and trust that we will be led down the right road.

*With the help of my Higher Power,
I receive the guidance I need for decision-making
throughout my pregnancy.*

Date / /

Today I Feel

Fear Of Caring

Day 51

Children are such a precious gift to our world. As we progress in our pregnancy, we become more aware of children around us. We may find ourselves wondering if they have a safe, healthy and caring home life.

As mothers-to-be, we may have the urge to wrap our arms around every single child to protect them from harm. This feeling may be so overwhelming it frightens us. We need to trust that God is caring for the universe which includes all children.

*Caring about all children is natural at this time,
and as my own sense of motherhood grows,
I look forward to many peaceful
moments with my child.*

Date / /

Today I Feel _____

Courage

Day 52

Pregnancy is upon us: a decision we deliberated for months and a path we envisioned and prayed for. Now there is no turning back. What brought us here? What continues to lead us? What makes it possible for us to face labor and delivery? Courage!

We already have exemplified tremendous courage. Becoming pregnant and having this child is a very courageous act, especially for those who face it alone. We have mustered the confidence, the strength of spirit, willingness of body and trust in God's presence to await our child. With courage we can trust the universe and not be afraid to go forth.

*With courage I face inner fears
and find my way.*

Date   /   /

Today I Feel

Right Time?

Day 53

As a child, we may have dreamed of one day having a healthy, loving family. But maybe we have now become pregnant unexpectedly, too quickly or just not at the "right time." Our pregnancy is still new and we have not yet felt movement, so it all seems unreal. We cannot identify with this fetus as a person and we feel uncertain about our circumstances. This ambivalence is not uncommon to expectant mothers, but it will pass in the second trimester when we begin to feel flutters. We need to trust that our Higher Power knows the "right time" better than we do.

I must have faith, sometimes blind,
in my Higher Power to guide me lovingly
throughout my pregnancy.

Date / /

Today I Feel _____

Age

Day 54

Careers, travel, education or finances might be reasons why we did not have children in our twenties. Maybe we did not feel mature enough or did not want to be tied down. Whatever the reason, we can congratulate ourselves for having the wisdom to wait and not succumb to pressures.

Now, as an "older mother," we face a slightly higher risk of complications, but we do not face this alone. Our friends, family and obstetrician will all give us support. Also, we know that medical advances have greatly reduced the risks of having a baby late in life.

*I keep a positive mind about
this very natural event.*

Date   /   /

Today I Feel

Feeling Pulse

Day 55

How do I feel today? What if we start our day by taking a quick, five second check or, better yet, several checks throughout the day? How am I feeling? Do I need to eat something to avoid nausea? Am I feeling more emotional today? Tired?

Whatever our mood, by taking time to identify it, we can feel more in control. Also, we should gently remind ourselves that our hormones are acting differently during this time and we should try not to let this interfere with our plans.

When I feel the extreme moods of pregnancy, I remind myself that it's "only hormones." Even though they are real, they're also exaggerated now.

Date   /   /

Today I Feel

Growth

Day 56

Are we willing to try and grow by accepting risk? Are we dedicated to helping our partner grow and letting him help us? We may have been uncertain about having a family, but our partner has been encouraging us, and now we find ourselves pregnant.

We may not have felt one hundred percent ready to get pregnant, but with our partner's support, we have decided to have this child. He has seen the possibility for positive growth in sharing our love where we have not.

We continue to depend on him to help us get the care we need and also to deal with fears that creep in.

I feel grateful to have the concern and encouragement of my partner for this new venture.

Date / /

Today I Feel _____

Shadow

Day 57

Even though we are aware of the signs of co-dependency, we may temporarily find ourselves losing our way. There may be times during our pregnancy when we fall back into our old, familiar patterns, but we must not be too hard on ourselves. We know when we are under a lot of stress, "relapse" can occur.

Certainly pregnancy is both stressful and full of changes. Sometimes we feel as if others "get to us," taking us over. We need to be gentle with ourselves and accept that our Higher Power will guide us toward our highest good.

*I will continue to live my own life
with strength and independence in the interest
of the baby and myself.*

Date   /   /

Today I Feel

Resistance

Day 58

Our pregnancy may fall into the category of a surprise. If it was unplanned, we may be trying to sort out and possibly resist the change. Why would we fend off such a positive blessing?

One reason could be fear: of failure as a parent, of responsibility or of labor itself. Pushing us out of our comfort zones, fear can be disturbing. We may think, "Things were good in my life until now" or "Things were terrible and now they will be worse." We need to force ourselves out of our current thinking, identify our fears and leave them behind.

*The more I understand these changes,
and the fears that surround them, the easier it is
to accept this as an opportunity to grow.*

Date / /

Today I Feel

Struggle

Day 59

What a struggle some of us have when we first learn we are pregnant. We feel it is a mistake and wonder what its purpose is. We may feel alone and afraid, asking, "How could God let this happen to me?"

What if there were a way to feel hopeful, happy and peaceful? Wouldn't we want to investigate it? Many people claim it starts by acknowledging a power greater than ourselves. Turning our lives over to God, we can see a plan unfold that we are blind to right now.

It may seem difficult to give our struggle to God, but by letting our Higher Power handle our lives, we receive relief, grace and peace.

By declaring God an important aspect of my life,
I find it easier to see the goodness of my pregnancy.

Date / /

Today I Feel _____

Double Edge

Day 60

Many of us feel ecstatic that we are pregnant. It has taken years to get pregnant, we finally met the right person and our dream of having a child is finally happening. While we revel in this excitement, we also must acknowledge other feelings, such as sadness.

Why sadness at such a wonderful time? Because we know we are leaving behind another life. Deep down we know that in time we will adapt to our new treasure-filled life, but in the meantime we may need to let ourselves grieve a little for the loss of our present life.

I acknowledge grief as I let go of one part of my life and welcome the new.

Date / /

Today I Feel

Plan

Day 61

Praying for peace and health for ourselves, our family and our baby is not selfish, but a realization that what we have in our lives is part of a plan.

God has a plan for our lives and these gifts are not to be taken for granted. Asking for continued peace and health is only a way of saying we know our Higher Power is the source of our well-being. We recognize that we must trust that source for continued guidance.

Being under the unsleeping eye of the One who watches over us and our baby, day and night, assures us of everlasting care.

Higher Power, fill my heart with love and help me trust in your plan for my life.

Date / /

Today I Feel

Sibling Role

Day 62

Adding another member to a family can be very exciting. Older children anticipate a playmate, someone to share secrets with. They may be wondering how they will fill their new role as brother or sister and how this baby will affect their relationship with us.

We need to take an active role in preparing our children for the new arrival. Together we can look through their baby books, talk about their births and even share role play with their toys. These activities help prepare them for the baby. The more involved they are, the easier they will accept the new baby.

I will "get out of myself" by involving my other children in the preparations.

Date / /

Today I Feel _____

Manly Pride

Day 63

Ever since our partner learned we are pregnant, his "manly pride" seems to be in high gear. Is his excitement due to his discovery of his virility or is he happy about the coming child? In time this initial thrill will fade as the reality sinks in.

Although we may be obsessed with ourselves, we must not forget our partner's emotions. He, too, is a part of this, going through the nine months of changes and later sharing the experience of parenting. Together we have got into this experience, a team for pregnancy, birthing and parenting.

I try to pay attention to my partner's emotions, allowing him to participate in this as much as possible.

Date / /

Today I Feel

Patterns

Day 64

While pregnant we may develop new patterns of behavior that we need to be aware of. For instance, we may become extremely overtired. The first thing we tend to feel is irritable and begin taking it out on our partner and friends. As one woman said, "I start biting his head off for every little thing." When other people become targets or entangled in our behavioral patterns, we need to take some time to sort ourselves out. These lessons prepare us for motherhood which will bring out both the worst and the best.

Spending time sorting out my behavior helps me become the parent I want to be.

Date   /   /

Today I Feel

Loneliness

Day 65

Sometimes, unintentionally, we end up going in separate directions from our partners. Our lives, daily routines and priorities change and communication is lacking or shut off. This can happen because of our new direction and will continue changing once the baby is with us. Our individual priorities shift as we familiarize ourselves with new territories and responsibilities. Separate from each other, we feel detached and possibly are not the same team anymore. We feel like a dotted line and no longer a circle. If we are to parent together, however, the situation is one we need to work on.

I am never alone — God is with me at all times especially through my life transitions.

Date / /

Today I Feel _____

_____

_____

_____

Listening

Day 66

We may find ourselves curious about how other women have managed the experience of pregnancy. "How did Jan handle being pregnant, working full time and going to school?" "How did a scaredy cat like Sheila ever handle labor?" "How does Gail manage to have two kids and do everything else she does?"

By listening to others in similar circumstances we gain a sense of confidence and begin believing that we, too, can be successful. Stories of pregnancy and parenting provide us with strength. We will not feel as uncertain when we know this is a road others have traveled.

I draw tremendous strength from other women who have gone through this.

Date / /

Today I Feel

The Journey

Day 67

Long ago we may not have thought we wanted children. We swore that, no matter what, we would never bring a child into this world. Yet, here we are, wondering when those ideas left.

Somewhere along our journey we have changed. Our values are different and so is how we spend our time. We are more placid, self-contained, satisfied and comfortable. We know, too, that in our hearts nothing could be more right than having a child.

There's no telling how long this feeling will last. Enjoy it and remember it the next time we lie awake weeping in the dark.

I treasure these wonderful moments and remember them when I am feeling down.

Date / /

Today I Feel _____

The Night

Day 68

The night is a time for resting our tired bodies and minds. The night also can become an enemy, bringing fears and worries about our new status in life.

There are several things we can do to ensure the relaxing rest we need. First, we must try to resolve problems during the day and let them go at night. Second, we need relaxing activities such as our pre-bed routine. Last, we must remind ourselves that problems seem ten times worse during the night. Let them go. They will be there in the morning light.

I do my best to give myself the peaceful rest I need.

Date / /

Today I Feel

Self-Esteem

Day 69

We want our children to grow up with a healthy sense of self-esteem and confidence, comfortable with decision making and secure about their values and morals. To cultivate this successfully in our children, we need to look first at our family of origin.

Did we feel respected, cared for and important? Did we feel nurtured, loved and supported during our growing up years? Were we encouraged to show affection, be creative and talk about our fears? And were we admired for our individual strengths and given help with weaknesses?

As we prepare for the birth of our child, we need to look at our own family to see what we need to heal and what we wish to keep in our parenting.

> ***The main thing I need to do is believe in the goodness of myself and my baby.***

Date / /

Today I Feel _____

Privacy

Day 70

Throughout our lives we have valued our privacy. Some of us may feel shy about the lack of privacy we experience during pregnancy. Strangers talk to us, touch us or stare at us. Doctors poke, probe and examine. Nurses and other technicians ask endless questions. As difficult as all this is, some things cannot be changed and this may be one of them. Although we ought to be able to expect a certain respect, we probably can do little to change the fact that our privacy is temporarily lost. As soon as we accept this, we will become more at ease.

I try to understand the reasons why my privacy seems lost and learn ahead of time what routines to expect.

Date / /

Today I Feel _____

Sensitivity

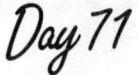

Day 71

In the next forty weeks we are going to feel emotions like never before. Our bodies are experiencing great fluctuations in hormone levels. We need to find medical advisors who are both medically competent and compassionate.

Do we have a good rapport with our obstetrician? Is the staff cordial? Is information shared willingly?

One of the responsibilities of pregnancy is finding a doctor who will meet all our needs. We should demand this kind of service because we are the customer. Too often we expect doctors to read our minds and we settle for less than what we need.

I am doing my best to develop a two-way trusting relationship with my doctor.

Date / /

Today I Feel

The Seed

Day 72

A seed is indeed a miraculous little thing. It can grow in almost any environment, whether in a forest, woods, backyard, crack of a sidewalk or pot on a windowsill. The only elements it needs to survive are water, air and sun.

In the same way, a seed has been planted within us. It, too, is struggling to survive, to become lush and to flourish. Our bodies are its protection. We are the sunshine, air and rain, the sole providers for this seed. It is up to us to nurture it well.

Nature will take its course in developing my baby,
but I must remember my responsibility in nourishing it.

Date / /

Today I Feel

Childhood Ending

Day 73

We are truly becoming adults now, no matter what our age may be. The experience of having a child of our own puts a final end to our childhood. We, too, will be parents, just like our parents and grandparents. This role symbolizes an ending, but also a new beginning full of adventures and responsibilities. We move on to a new identity.

Feeling comfortable with our new role as a parent takes patience and courage. We can't just let go of our present identity in exchange for another. It takes time to learn our new tasks as we leave childhood and enter into adulthood.

*Letting go of childhood is sad, but I know
I am entering a whole new world
that is fun and challenging.*

Date / /

Today I Feel _____

Risk

Day 74

How do we feel about risk? A common reaction is fear. We may look upon our pregnancy as taking a risk and naturally feel a little fearful.

But we need to think about the reality of this risk. What is real and what is only perceived?

While rock climbing on a mountainside, we may be scared being thousands of feet in the air with only sharp rocks around us. We know that if we fall, we could die. As soon as we remember the two safety ropes tied to us, we can see this is a "perceived risk" and enjoy the gorgeous scenery.

*I need to take care of any real risks,
finding my "safety ropes" in those around
me and in my Higher Power.*

Date / /

Today I Feel

Worry

Day 75

Most of us do our share of worrying during pregnancy because there is a lot to be concerned about. Will the baby be healthy? Will we have enough money? What has happened to our sex life? How will my job be affected?

Our minds are preoccupied with planning for the arrival, but also trying to deal with fatigue and nausea.

If worry is draining us of energy, we need to evaluate our concerns. What are we truly worried about? Our network of family and friends can help us by offering guidance and reminding us that we are not in this alone.

I alleviate the stress of worry with the help of my partner, friends, doctor and Higher Power.

Date / /

Today I Feel

Tests

Day 76

Many diagnostic tests are now routinely prescribed to rule out problems during early pregnancy: ultrasound, alpha fetoprotein and amniocentesis. The chance of a problem is slim, but if something is wrong, we need to know early.

If a problem is found, we need to research these tests together with our partner, meet with medical advisors and get involved in genetic counseling. We will then be able to make an informed decision about this pregnancy. We are not in this alone because we can trust in our Higher Power to help us with our choices.

Through education I learn to comfort my doubts, and my Higher Power helps me come to the right decisions.

Date / /

Today I Feel _____

_____

_____

_____

Sexual Honesty

Day 77

Sex is such a wonderful way of expressing love with our partner, a beautiful way to feel close. Our baby is a product of this love and our commitment to build a family, a future and a home.

During pregnancy, our attitude about sex may change. We don't respond the way we used to. We may not be interested or we lack energy. Or we feel self-conscious. What can we do to relieve this?

We need to reassure our husbands of our love, but not fake physical or mental feeling. In the long run, fake responses only lead to alienation and dishonesty.

My life is different now and that includes sex,
but I feel assured it is only temporary.

Date / /

Today I Feel _____

Responsibility

Day 78

Responsibility increases as life progresses. As infants, we had no responsibilities and were dependent on others. As children, we had few responsibilities other than chores or homework. As we approached adolescence, independence increased with our first job, getting a driver's license or babysitting.

With each year of adulthood, more complicated responsibilities appear: marriage, mortgage, taxes and career. Having a baby adds one more.

Parenthood will require us to put our baby's needs first. This responsibility is most important and will change over the years as our child grows.

I know the responsibility of a child will add an exciting challenge to my daily life.

Date / /

Today I Feel _____

Mom's "Curse"

Day 79

We all remember hearing, "You just wait till you have your own daughter!" Now, as expectant mothers, we may be trying to figure out what we'll be getting back twofold from this little creature developing inside us.

Our current situation prompts us to reflect on our relationship with our own mother. What did we like, dislike, love, hate? What did we find comfort and security in? On the other hand, what did we do to bring sorrow, joy or happiness to her? Becoming a parent is an excellent time to forgive our mother and ourselves, and establish a greater love between us.

The experiences with my mother are guidance for raising my own child.

Date   /   /

Today I Feel _____

_____

_____

_____

Guilt

Day 80

An expectant mother wakes up one morning extremely tired from a night of dancing. Although she didn't drink or smoke, she did stay out late and now she has little energy, but lots of guilt.

Why the guilt? She really did nothing wrong, but in her mind she thinks a pregnant woman should stay home and knit booties. Even though this image is far from her lifestyle, she still accepts it. We need to continue having fun, not abuse ourselves for still being ourselves. As long as we're responsible about our pregnancy, whatever we choose to do is fine.

As long as I am taking good care of myself and the baby, I refuse to feel guilty for not being a "typical" pregnant woman.

Date / /

Today I Feel _____

Support Team

Day 81

Our pregnancy is a long journey, but one we do not travel alone. This is a great time to establish our support team. First we need a doctor whose medical awareness and compassion we feel comfortable with. Then we need to think about a coach for childbirth, someone we feel completely at ease with. And last, we need to develop a network of other support people. A friend who is also pregnant is great to communicate with on a regular basis. How about neighbors or family? They can all become part of our network, a team of people to support us during our pregnancy.

Each individual in my network has different strengths which combine to make a stronger backbone than my own, alone.

Date   /   /

Today I Feel _____

_____

_____

Steps

Day 82

We let go of a lot of stress when we try to take our pregnancy one day at a time. We focus our energy on today, not worries of tomorrow or concerns of yesterday. But even then there can be problems.

Sometimes the steps we take today may not turn out to be the best, although we had that intention. Even if we alter our diet to avoid health problems, we may still retain water and swell up.

We cannot look ahead and know for certain that the steps we are taking today will be the right ones, but we need to have the courage to make a good effort. Above all, we must have trust in our Higher Power to guide us.

*Just as my baby will one day,
I take one step at a time.*

Date / /

Today I Feel _____

Relaxation

Day 83

Let us take time to sit back in the quiet and close our eyes. So much of our energy is going toward taking care of our jobs, family and household that we easily neglect to give attention to ourselves. Ordinary relaxation seems to disappear. In order to give all these other areas of our lives the quality of attention they need (and expect), we must first give it to ourselves. Sitting in the quiet, relaxing and concentrating only on our breathing, gives us the break needed to recharge our batteries.

*Today I remember to take time out
for simple relaxation. I need quality time for
myself in order to give it to others.*

Date / /

Today I Feel _____

Seesaw

Day 84

Another day has come and gone. As we reflect upon its events, we may feel as if we have been on an emotional seesaw. Nothing seems normal. Our reactions and thoughts make no sense to us. "What is going on?" we wonder.

We just need to let go as we pass through this transitory stage of hormonal changes. We must let this day go and understand that we cannot control it. Tomorrow is a new dawn. We deserve peace of mind, rest and a new start. We must be gentle with ourselves and find hope in the knowledge that everything passes.

I accept the emotional seesaw I am on and realize that by letting go I will find freedom to receive the present and future.

Date / /

Today I Feel _____

Myths

Day 85

When we are pregnant, everyone seems to offer us their favorite bit of advice: "You're carrying low, it's a boy." "This is your first baby? Oh, you'll deliver late. Always early on the second." "Your father was a twin? You'll probably have twins." "Aren't you glad this is your third? Your labor will be a breeze!" The most important thing we can do is ask our doctor what truth, if any, is behind these helpful comments. We can also develop patience and chuckle at our sudden popularity. Unfortunately, pregnancy makes us vulnerable to frequent comments and advice.

I work on keeping my sense of humor, vital in these nine months and the years ahead.

Date / /

Today I Feel

Letters

Day 86

Writing to another person, keeping a journal or diary, or starting a baby book is an excellent way of communicating with others. We share our feelings and we record important events. And we create a keepsake for the baby. So often through our nine months we feel overwhelmed with emotions. It is important that we release them in a healthy manner. By writing, we get them off our minds. Finding creative ways to vent concerns can be a fun process. It will be interesting later to see how we felt when we were pregnant, when it is such a fleeting time in our lives overall.

When my emotions mount, I write them down as a healthy way to have a hold on my feelings, before they get a hold on me!

Date   /   /

Today I Feel _____

_____

_____

_____

Physical Changes

Day 87

Things may be happening to our bodies that we may not understand. We have tried to ask our doctor all our questions, but that just doesn't seem like enough.

Sometimes we need more, some kind of a reference book to have nearby to answer concerns that come up at odd moments. Our friends can't answer all our questions and some of the experiences we are having may be different than theirs. Our mothers know a lot about having babies, but the experience is different now. By finding a good reference guide at a library, clinic, friend or doctor, we build confidence in ourselves.

I find the resources I need so that I may feel at ease in my pregnancy.

Date / /

Today I Feel _____

Flexibility

Day 88

During our pregnancy we will relieve a lot of stress if we try to remain flexible. If we are too rigid, we may find it hard to cope when outside factors change our plans. This is reflected in our daily schedules, appointments with our doctor and how we get along with our husbands.

We may have had expectations in the past, but now it's time for us to learn that spontaneity has a place in our plans. Rather than fighting change, we need to realize that "life happens." Learning to be flexible now will prepare us for when the baby arrives. Flexibility is mandatory for staying sane with a newborn.

I will try to "go with the flow" and not impose my will on life so much.

Date / /

Today I Feel

Grandparents

Day 89

Each of us has different types of grandparents for our child. When thinking about their role in our child's life, we need to be realistic and honest.

We begin by reflecting on our relationship with them. How were we treated as children? Is there mutual love and respect? Do we value their presence in our lives? Are they thrilled by the baby? Do they make us feel apprehensive?

Whatever our feelings, it is important to consider this now because our child will sense how we feel. We need to be honest about the role we see the grandparents playing in our child's life.

I take a serious look at the role of grandparents in my baby's life and talk with them about any concerns I have.

Date / /

Today I Feel _____

Dreams

Day 90

Dreams of our future are significant for enriching our lives. First we dream, then we make it come true.

Our baby is part of a dream we had long ago, a dream of the future. And here we are, in what was once part of our future.

Some dreams are meant to come true. What dreams do we have now for the future of this baby? College, health, athletic achievement, fame? The way to achieve these dreams is by planning, but also by instilling positive self-esteem in our child.

*The most important role I will play as a parent
is helping my children see themselves in a positive light.
All children are gifted individuals with the
ability to make a difference.*

Date / /

Today I Feel _____

_____

_____

_____

Heartbeat

Day 91

Ambivalence describes how we feel toward our developing baby. We are excited that we are pregnant, but it doesn't seem real yet, which makes us uneasy. Shouldn't we be feeling overwhelming love? But how can we, when we have not seen it, felt it or heard it? Our body has gone through some changes, but nothing really feels too different. Rest assured that all uncertainty will leave when we hear our baby's heartbeat for the first time. Our doctor can amplify the sound so we do not think we are just imagining things. We will always remember this as a special moment.

My baby becomes much more real to me once I hear the heartbeat, the sweet music to my ears.

Date / /

Today I Feel _____

Criticism

Day 92

We know our husband cares very much about us and the healthy development of our child. From time to time in the pregnancy, he may make some suggestions. We can more easily accept this if we realize his efforts are sincere. His support can actually be a kind of saving grace.

Sometimes, though, too much can turn us off. Occasionally bringing work home or having a sip of a beer does not deserve constant criticism. If he watches our every move, waiting to catch us doing something wrong, our supportive relationship may be turning sour. With communication and help from our Higher Power, we can put this team back on balance.

I will talk to my husband and communicate my concerns. We both have a vested interest in "our" pregnancy.

Date / /

Today I Feel

Late Life Baby

Day 93

Due to medical reasons, we had been told that our chances of having a baby were slim. But now, much older than the average expectant mother, we are on cloud nine!

Unfortunately, our spouse may not be as excited. He may feel he is set in his ways, too old to be a father and afraid of this change. Just when our lives are starting to feel complete, our husband's commitment to having a child may be wavering. We need to get him to talk with us and remind him that he, too, has forty weeks to get used to this idea. We are in this together and we need him to work with us.

*Together my spouse and I
can make this work
and welcome a beautiful child.*

Date / /

Today I Feel

Non-Gravity

Day 94

Movement within is extremely comforting to any expectant mother. Once we start feeling it, we get used to it and look forward to it. What a thrill and a natural high. Movement tells us that our baby is healthy and thriving in our womb.

At certain times during the day, our baby seems more active. After eating certain foods we may notice a definite period of activity. Or when we finally put our feet up at the end of a long day, our babies may decide to act up. As our babies grow and develop, their movements become more frequent and stronger, floating around in this gravity-free world.

*My baby is already working
on developing coordination skills,
a miracle in the making.*

Date / /

Today I Feel

Second Trimester

Comfort Zone

Day 95

For so long, we have been living within a "comfort zone," the same activities, social events and routines — not having to face change. We have spent hours at the office, weekends at our PCs and holidays working at home. Whatever our pattern, it is being permanently disrupted by having a baby.

This new adventure will certainly be challenging, although we may feel threatened by all this change. Comfort zones are hard to give up!

We need to accept these changes that bring growth and new experiences. Our lives will never be the same!

*Whether I was satisfied with my routines or not,
I open my heart and life to the changes that are coming.*

Date / /

Today I Feel

Crying

Day 96

What better way to cleanse our mind and body than to have a good cry? Letting emotions build up is bad for us at any time in our lives. Sometimes the best way to feel better is simply to let ourselves cry when we feel like it, which seems much easier to do now. We may cry because we feel overwhelmed or we may not be able to pinpoint the reason.

Before we got pregnant, we may have rarely shed tears, but now it seems as if they flow easily. Our lives have changed, our hormones are imbalanced and crying is a natural reaction to trying to cope. There is nothing wrong with this and we need to be gentle with ourselves.

*Crying is common and healthy,
nature's way of helping me to cleanse my mind and body.*

Date / /

Today I Feel

Coach's Role

Day 97

There are many benefits to having a coach throughout our pregnancy, and especially during labor and delivery. This person becomes real support for us, sharing the experience. He or she takes childbirth classes with us and is there when we need a good friend.

A coach can be anyone: spouse, friend, parent or sibling. All that matters is that this person is dependable and we trust them. The role of coach is also very spiritual. They help us build confidence in ourselves, giving us extra energy, encouraging words and a sense of humor when we most need it.

I spend some time thinking about who would be a good coach for my birthing experience.

Date / /

Today I Feel _____

Past Power

Day 98

Shame and guilt are two very destructive feelings, emotional baggage from our past. We all have done things we regret and can't forget. The memory creeps up on us, sometimes when we least expect it, leaving us feeling anxious. While we are pregnant, these memories throw us off balance when we want to be happy. However, a trusted friend or counselor can help us put our fears to rest and assure us that the past is gone. Our medical advisors can answer questions about how past experiences may affect the baby. Making use of the resources around us, we find greater peace in our pregnancy.

When I feel anxious about the past, I am grateful I can seek out the support of my Higher Power and my close friends.

Date / /

Today I Feel _____

_____

_____

_____

Lecturing

Day 99

Much needs to be discussed during these weeks, from diaper service to names. But when we excitedly start talking with our partner about "baby stuff," he responds, "Oh boy, another lecture." Our excitement turns to anger and we clam up. What went wrong? Could we be guilty of lecturing?

Lecturing is primarily a conversation that is one-sided. We talk and do not let up. We are constantly telling instead of allowing give and take. We need to find ways to communicate "with" our partners and friends, not "at."

*I will find ways to relate better
or I won't have the support I need.*

Date   /   /

Today I Feel _____

Big Breasted

Day 100

In addition to the unpleasant side effects, such as swollen feet, varicose veins and weight gain, we also may develop larger breasts. For many of us, this may seem like a dream come true.

Soon enough we realize the downside to large breasts. Males may not know how to react to such a phenomenon, evident in jokes and stares. This type of behavior makes us feel objectified and uncomfortable. Our circumstances do not make us public property, as normally large-breasted women must feel every day of their lives.

*Physical changes are my own to experience and
I do not have to put up with rudeness,
although I am also learning to ignore
some of this unwanted attention.*

Date / /

Today I Feel _____

Angel Wings

Day 101

Exhilarating describes the first fetal movements we experience. Just when we think we will never feel anything, we are caught by surprise by a fluttering that leaves behind the most wonderful feelings. Finally our pregnancy seems real. Angel wings will continue to flutter about inside of us from this day forward. Soon, in this trimester, others will also be able to see and feel these movements. This will make the pregnancy seem more real to them as they feel their future son, grandchild or sister. Everyone will feel so much closer to this experience and more confident. We will continue to be surprised as our baby kicks out when we're in a budget meeting, in a restaurant, doing the dishes or trying to sleep.

I thank my Higher Power each night for this wonderful gift.

Date   /   /

Today I Feel _____

Chronic Uncertainty

Day 102

Where is the woman we used to be? Once we were confident and competent, but now we are insecure and indecisive. Before we always knew where we were going, but now we feel lost, like a small child again.

Pregnancy is a new experience with its own agenda. We may easily feel insecure when faced with weird physical sensations and unknown emotions. This experience may be overwhelming, especially if we are handling it alone.

> *Any uncertainty is offset by depending on the support of other pregnant friends, my family, doctor and Higher Power.*

Date / /

Today I Feel _____

Natural Child

Day 103

For many, this may be our second or third child, but the first with this husband. We are very excited to be pregnant again because the time seems right. Our husband has been great with our other children. We cannot help but wonder, though, if he may favor this child because it will be his own.

We need not waste time being concerned about this, but we must talk with our husband. He will naturally have a different love, a different connection with this child, but that is all it will be. In many ways this baby will help to bring our family closer.

*I don't keep concerns like this inside,
but talk them over with my spouse
and come to understanding and peace.*

Date / /

Today I Feel _____

Burnout

Day 104

Heavy involvement in a job, plus community and home responsibilities, may drive us to burnout. The symptoms are varied: exhaustion, apathy or insomnia.

Being pregnant means we have to reduce our activities by learning to say no. We need to evaluate our lives and get back to basics such as eating, sleeping and relaxing. Burnout will only lead to desperation and possible health problems. We need to do what we can to avoid it throughout our pregnancy.

A pregnancy is less than two percent of an average lifetime. Why must I do everything now? Is it really important enough to risk the health of my baby and myself?

Date / /

Today I Feel _____

Acceptance

Day 105

We all know some women who are unable to get pregnant or to carry a baby to term. We may feel guilty and resist sharing our excitement. We realize it must be painful for them to witness our joy and fulfillment. We can, however, show our compassion by sharing the sorrow they must feel.

We can also pray they find the strength to accept their reality and that maybe it will change. Deep in our hearts, we know life progresses according to God's loving plan for all of us. There is a rightness to what happens to all of us in life, whether we can perceive it or not at the time.

If I commit my life to God, my purpose remains steady and fulfilling, no matter what circumstances I encounter.

Date / /

Today I Feel

Logic

Day 106

Sometimes we act before we think, which can be hurtful to others, especially little ones. Instead of just reacting, we need to walk away and think about the situation. If we acted at work the way we do at home, some of us wouldn't have jobs!

Why does such conflict happen? The answer now is partly hormones, although at any stage of our lives, we need lessons like this. Being aware of our tendency to fly off the handle is a step in the right direction. We can work on improving our communication, ask for forbearance and recognize the ways we do succeed.

*I try to be more logical and less reactive
in my relationships. But when I fail, I can forgive
myself and improve next time.*

Date / /

Today I Feel

Personal Worth

Day 107

Do we want our child to grow up happy, successful and optimistic? Of course we do. Then we need to be aware of one particular ingredient: self-esteem. To help our child have a healthy personality, we need to cultivate a positive sense of self-worth.

We start with love, the most important human gift. From today on, we can foster this feeling. The baby will sense it by the sound of our voice, the touch of our hands and the jiggling of our laughter. Once he joins us in the world, he will be surrounded by the love in our reactions, the reflection in our eyes and softness of our touch. Together we can achieve positive self-worth.

The gift of love is so beautiful, already growing between us and our child.

Date / /

Today I Feel _____

Shame

Day 108

Shame can leave us feeling empty and sad. It is so easy to say things we don't mean, especially when we are tired. We may lash out in anger: "You don't care about this baby at all! You're going to make a terrible father!"

During pregnancy, we may behave in a shameful manner without intending to. When our partner is having an emotional crisis, instead of helping, we blame him for not meeting our expectations. We must remember that our partner is also experiencing adjustment and in need of understanding. After speaking hurtful words, the best recourse is asking forgiveness.

*I more easily find peace if I am
gentle with those I love.*

Date / /

Today I Feel _____

Tools

Day 109

Think about what it would be like to build a treehouse without a saw, fix a leaky faucet without a wrench or put up dry wall without a tape measure. We can't repair, create or build without the proper tools. In the same way, we need to make sure we have the right tools to help us with this pregnancy.

Tools are all around us, helping us perform well and achieve our goals. Resources are important tools, such as our doctor or health books. Vitamins and nutritious food are tools to help us be strong. Our body is our ultimate tool that helps us design and build the most intricate creation in the world.

__Do I have the right tools to assist me to reach my goals during pregnancy?__

Date / /

Today I Feel _____

Time

Day 110

Moment by moment, time just keeps slipping by. There will be occasions when we turn inward and question the direction of our lives. "What if I hadn't done this or that? Where would I be now? And where am I going now that I'm becoming a mother?"

We wish we could just put a stop to time but it is not a living thing. Time simply exists, moment by moment, ticking away.

Picture yourself as a bird, free in the air, flying through clouds and over mountains. Time does not exist in nature. You keep flying once your baby comes, not worried, but flying through change, growth, challenge and joy alongside this new person.

Life goes on all around me, and soon I will have a new friend to share it with.

Date / /

Today I Feel _____

Twelve Steps

Day 111

Various emotional struggles come with being pregnant. Many of us have found strength in the past through the Twelve Steps of Alcoholics Anonymous or other support groups. We know we can now depend on the Twelve Steps to support us through this time. We can apply this program to our pregnancy and adopt the principles to our present needs.

The Twelve Steps can give us support, help us put the past behind us and let our Higher Power direct our lives. They can enable us to sort out our lives to become the parent we want to be.

Now in unfamiliar territory, I find great peace from the Twelve Steps to promote spiritual wellness.

Date / /

Today I Feel _____

Emotional Pain

Day 112

How much emotional pain are we experiencing these days? Do we find ourselves running from it because it is too unbearable? Are we denying it because we want to keep up the image of the perfectly happy expectant mother? The only remedy is to identify the pain, although it is a lot harder now that our lives are so complicated.

First we need to look at our lives: finances, health, relationship, work. What is bringing stress into our lives?

By acknowledging what is causing us pain, we can seek relief and begin to feel more hopeful about our lives.

Neglecting emotional pain will only get me stuck and stressed out, so I give some time to confronting it.

Date / /

Today I Feel _____

Voices

Day 113

How many times do we hear a little voice inside us instilling fear and worry? Do we succumb to that voice? Or do we tell it to go away and leave us alone? Each time we hear this voice, we need to dismiss it.

If the voice brings up health concerns, we counter with our latest good checkup. If the voice tells us to go ahead and pick up three laundry baskets or stand on a chair to reach a high shelf, we need to respond with a quick no! If the voice starts to bring up how painful delivery will be, we answer, "I am strong. I am doing everything to prepare myself. I will take one contraction at a time."

Each time I silence the derogatory voice,
I become stronger and the voice becomes weaker,
eventually fading away.

Date / /

Today I Feel _____

_____

_____

_____

Sex

Day 114

"Where do babies come from? How does it get in there?" We are certain to hear such questions from preschoolers at home or in our neighborhoods. Pregnancy is a complicated topic for young children to comprehend and their curiosity is natural.

We can let peers or the media later tell our children about sex and childbirth, hoping they receive the information they need. Or we can involve ourselves in this effort. Truly our children will benefit if we share information with them. What better time to talk together about this important topic?

With the help of my spouse and my Higher Power, I trust that I will help my children develop a healthy attitude about sex.

Date / /

Today I Feel _____

Shutting Out

Day 115

Listening to our family and friends is so important. If we are interrupting or distracted while they are talking, we are not giving them our total attention. If we are shutting them out a lot lately, we need to ask ourselves why. At this time in our lives, we need to be close to those around us, particularly our husbands.

First of all, how are others listening to us? Do they give us their undivided attention or do they watch TV? If this is happening, then maybe we don't pay attention because we think they don't deserve it. Now is the time to become better listeners, before we become parents.

*I am evaluating my listening skills
and thinking about ways to improve them.*

Date / /

Today I Feel _____

Roller Coaster

Day 116

We may find ourselves acting in ways we never have before. Our partner may be the recipient of outbursts or constant edginess. On the other hand, he himself may be acting as if nothing has changed. He may not be supporting us in the ways we need at this time.

The coming child will have great impact on our relationship. We prepare for this with the ups and downs of pregnancy. We are undoubtedly facing parenting with trepidation since it can seem scary. These new roles will continue to take us along life's roller coaster.

*Through good communication with those I love,
I feel more trust at a time when negative
emotions can easily be triggered.*

Date / /

Today I Feel _____

New Life/New Hope

Day 117

We have chosen to offer a home to a new person. This is truly a blessing in our lives. Our baby is a direct reflection of the love we have for our husband and our Higher Power. This blessing is also a reflection of our Higher Power's love for us.

We have received a gift, one we will spend hours watching in awe and cradling in our arms, wondering what the future holds. We pray that there will be good in our world, beauty in our days and significance in our efforts. By sharing our human love, we are renewing our faith in the promise of tomorrow.

The growing life within me constantly reminds me of my commitment to marriage, family and faith in the future.

Date / /

Today I Feel _____

Normalcy

Day 118

To have our lives feel "normal" right now is an impossibility because we are experiencing so many changes. There really is not a normal day, week or even hour. Our way of life may seem completely disrupted, but in reality we are right on target.

As we experience change in our lives, our sense of what normalcy is also changes. Once things become more stabilized, a new definition of normal exists. For us, this will be evolving constantly for quite some time as we head into parenting.

I take care not to get riled up about feeling that my life is not "normal" right now. I am restored and renewed even in the midst of change.

Date / /

Today I Feel _____

Checkups

Day 119

Poked and prodded may best describe our doctor's checkups, routines that can start to seem bothersome. Weight checks, blood tests and ultrasound, every month there's something new to check. Throughout we need to have a positive attitude because tests are only meant to help.

These procedures are all forms of measurement, the only way to tell how we are doing. By treating them as helpful tools, we are saying we trust them to keep us on track.

These measurements also help spot complications early. Our doctor can compare test results and keep us and our babies healthy.

I know measurement is necessary and plays an important role in my pregnancy.

Date / /

Today I Feel _____

Stubbornness

Day 120

Stubbornness can be difficult under the best of circumstances, but even harder while we are pregnant. We may become more stubborn as each day passes. Most likely it is all related to the lack of control we are feeling.

We are trying to handle so many changes that a natural coping method is to become less flexible and say, "This is the way it is, no ifs, ands or buts!" We feel we must remain in control of something.

We have stubbornly made up our minds about certain decisions and may not want to budge. By not giving in on small decisions, we feel we are gaining back control, but is it worth the loss of agreement with those we love?

*Stubbornness creates walls between people
and I want peace more than this.*

Date / /

Today I Feel _____

Partner

Day 121

Our minds can become obsessed with our pregnancy and all the tasks we have to handle. It is very easy to make family secondary. Granted, at times our spouse has to take a back seat to the priority at hand. However, if we continue to do this, our closeness will diminish and it won't be there when we need to depend on it later.

Our spouse deserves special attention during an emotional time like this. Time set aside to spend with him helps to keep our lines of communication open, resentments from growing and the love burning. Being appreciative also helps our relationship prosper. We want an environment where love flows freely and warmly — a perfect place for a baby.

A loving marriage creates a loving family.

Date / /

Today I Feel

Stress

Day 122

Being pregnant is an experience that makes us more vulnerable to stress. The best antidote is prevention.

Getting a good night's sleep, followed by breakfast, is the best way to start the day. We need short breaks during the day and we need to do something fun often. If we have difficulty accomplishing this, we simply have to say "stop" before ill health forces us to stop.

Affection also counteracts the build up of stress. Cuddling, hugging or simply holding hands promotes security and specialness. This helps relieve our stress and rechannels the energy.

Instead of taking things too seriously, I sit back, take time to laugh and listen to the raindrops.

Date / /

Today I Feel _____

Losing A Loved One

Day 123

Losing a loved one is difficult at any time, but can feel overwhelming during pregnancy. We can't stop crying, feel lonely and empty and angry that we did not get the chance to say goodbye.

Our unborn child will not have the chance to know this person who meant so much to us. Our baby will only know them through our stories and pictures. We pray that one day, too, our children will have a special person in their lives.

We should give ourselves special treatment during this emotionally draining time. We need to pay close attention to body signals to ensure we get the rest and nutrition we need.

Experiencing the loss of a loved one is particularly difficult now so I give myself extra attention and care. Never before have I felt the dichotomy between life and death so deeply.

Date / /

Today I Feel _____

_____

_____

_____

Gender

Day 124

Ultrasound tests during pregnancy can tell us the sex of our baby. As we lie on the table, the technician slides the applicator around and asks, "Would you like to know the sex? It's 99% accurate." Our hands start to sweat and our heart beats faster as we ponder our response. We thought we were committed to not finding out and preserving the mystery. After all, wouldn't it be more exciting to wait?

Now it just seems too easy. The pragmatic side takes over as we think about buying girl's clothes or decorating a boy's room. If we tend to be traditionalists, we might rather wait.

Finding out the sex of my child is up to my spouse and me; whatever we decide is right for us.

Date / /

Today I Feel _____

Healthy Environment

Day 125

Some individuals believe that violence is an acceptable way of dealing with conflict. This mindset is unhealthy, particularly when conflict occurs in the environment of a pregnant woman.

We are not only responsible for our own health but also that of our unborn child. If we're in a place that is violent, we need to move elsewhere for the benefit of ourselves and the baby. Many support groups and local agencies can help us make this difficult but imperative decision.

I take the responsibility to set limits on how others treat me to ensure that my baby and I are safe.

Date / /

Today I Feel _____

Vision

Day 126

When we go through a rough time in our lives, there is a lot of pain, suffering and fear. One thing that helps us through is vision. Vision is being able to look into the future and see the positive. We sense the things that make us happy, the goals we can achieve and the people we cherish. Vision helps give us the spark we need while taking one day at a time.

We also need to remember that low points in our lives are temporary. Soon we will have high points that are sweet and more peaceful again. Our pregnancy may have been part of a vision from our past, which is now filling us with positive feeling.

My Higher Power gives me the gift of vision and guides me at all times, good and bad.

Date / /

Today I Feel _____

Preparation

Day 127

It is the middle of the second trimester already and we still have a lot to do before the baby comes. There doesn't seem to be enough time for work, friends, family and preparing!

We need to remember the tools we have to help us. One of the simplest is a list, which can relieve us of having to remember everything. Post the list or keep it in your purse. Review it periodically and plan how you can accomplish these projects.

Remember also that friends and family can help. By sharing our needs with others, there is less burden and more time to enjoy this period in our lives.

To conserve energy and keep tasks in perspective, I will keep an ongoing list and ask others to help.

Date / /

Today I Feel _____

The Name Game

Day 128

For some, nine months is not long enough to come up with a name for our newest family member. We spend hours looking through name books and family trees, making lists and checking out name meanings.

Others may wait until the baby is born to see if she or he looks like a "Celia," a "John" or a "Sara." Some are pressured by family members to name the baby after a grandparent.

What seems simple turns quickly into a complicated process with pressure from everyone. A name is important, a lifelong label by which society will judge this new person.

> *I do not defer to others in making this decision;*
> *it is up to my spouse and me to name our baby.*

Date   /   /

Today I Feel _____

Letting Go

Day 129

Just when we think we can't go on another day, there is one last effort we can make that will save us: turning our pregnancy over to the care of our Higher Power. This will take care of our fears and concerns. True, we can continue struggling with our fears of parenting or unhappiness with our weight gain, but soon we realize that we can't control everything, all the time. Our pregnancy, and everyone involved with it, is beyond our control. Our bodies are in automatic mode of operation. Why not turn this over to the care of our Higher Power? This presence is always close to us, aware of our needs and providing unconditional love, no matter how cranky we get. Our Higher Power will be caring for us every day throughout our pregnancy.

I need to remember to let go and let God.

Date / /

Today I Feel _____

Caretaking

Day 130

If we already have children, we know what it is like to care for them. The hours we spend doing things for others are immeasurable. When we have our new baby, our caretaking will increase tremendously. Our days and nights will be consumed by changing diapers, feedings and doing laundry.

We need to watch out that our caring for others does not leave out care for ourselves. Although we can't neglect our families, we need to find little ways to nourish ourselves each day. Perhaps a few minutes alone with tea in the morning or a quiet bubble bath late at night.

My stamina is less now, but I still can find ways to take care of others and myself. The more care I give myself, the more care I can give others.

Date / /

Today I Feel

Love

Day 131

As our pregnancy develops, so does love for our unborn child. It's an overwhelming feeling we can't fully describe. We find ourselves becoming a different person in some ways, with more energy, hope and joy. We feel connected with people around us like never before. This deep emotion can be all-encompassing and it's just the beginning!

We are only in the second trimester with the third around the corner and the birth to follow. Our love feels like a warm hug with the whole world. When our baby arrives and throughout its growing years, our love will continue to grow.

I bask in the light of the love I feel for my child,
a special bond that will last a lifetime.

Date / /

Today I Feel _____

Fetal Movement

Day 132

Sitting in a restaurant or driving the car, we experience the first real movements of our baby. At first, we may have thought it was cramps or hunger, but soon there is no mistaking the strong fluttering fetal movements.

This is a sign that our baby is thriving and it affirms the new life within us. Every kick against our ribs or elbow in our side reminds us how wonderful the mystery of life truly is. This strong healthy person is forming itself with the help of our good care and the help of our Higher Power.

The simple, yet miraculous, feeling of fetal movement brings me joy throughout my pregnancy. I will savor this activity as a source of inner peace.

Date / /

Today I Feel

Baby's Father

Day 133

Today I am aware that my partner is thinking seriously about his changing role. Becoming a father means his life will change in many ways. He is taking on greater responsibility financially and emotionally, and perhaps he wonders how he'll handle it. This special man deserves understanding and appreciation as much as I do. We need to keep lines of communication open so that we can solve our problems together. It's more important than ever to keep our relationship healthy and strong. The future of our family depends on keeping love, honesty and harmony alive between us.

I will make it a point to keep our relationship loving and harmonious. Both of us deserve support.

Date / /

Today I Feel _____

Walking

Day 134

Taking care of ourselves physically during our pregnancy is very important. Have we given enough thought to exercise?

Walking on a daily basis reduces stress and gives us time to gather our thoughts. This time can be a meditation to review our day, our goals and our latest moods. It is a gift to ourselves and our baby. The rhythm of walking puts our baby to sleep or wakes it up. The stimulation is good for both of us. Walking helps to alleviate lower back pain, leg cramps, improves circulation and strengthens pelvic muscles. Mentally and physically, Mom and baby benefit.

I give my body the physical attention it deserves and enjoy the resulting peace.

Date   /   /

Today I Feel _____

Sacrifice

Day 135

The new lullaby of motherhood may be one of the best things to happen to us, but it does increase our responsibilities. We will find ourselves having to make sacrifices when we have children; there is only so much time in a day. Our jobs may take on less importance, but we may also feel more fulfilled in our life plan. Some job settings are more accommodating now, so we may be able to modify work to suit our family's needs. We may even decide not to be on the career track anymore. We may choose to work part-time or run a business at home. For many, there aren't options, with the financial realities of raising a child, but somewhere, somehow, we will find the right balance.

I will find the right path for me and my family in terms of work and income.

Date / /

Today I Feel _____

Anger

Day 136

How do we deal with anger? Do we suppress it? Express it? Accept it? Are others around us letting anger fester within them? Negative emotions are a part of life, not something we can hide from.

In our pregnancy it is important to confront our anger. We need to find ways to acknowledge it, feel it and take healthy action against it. We want to keep destructive emotions to a minimum so we do not find ourselves under stress that can affect our health. If not dealt with, anger can steal away the peace that is so important for us now.

I discuss this with my spouse and take healthy measures to deal with it.

Date / /

Today I Feel _____

Genetic Blueprint

Day 137

The genetic blueprint of our baby is established at conception. Although we may wish for a little boy who looks like our spouse, we may have one who looks more like bald Uncle Fred. We must also keep in mind that our baby's looks will change constantly, from the first moment we see them.

Having a healthy baby has to be foremost in the minds of all soon-to-be-parents, but our baby's appearance concerns us greatly. This process of genetics, a mystery to be enjoyed, will continue unfolding over years to come.

Fantasizing about my baby's looks is fun and meant to be enjoyed; however, a healthy baby is what I pray for.

Date / /

Today I Feel

Owning Feelings

Day 138

We experience a vast range of feelings while pregnant. Some may be new, some old and familiar. It is very important that we allow ourselves to "own" our feelings, not just experience them. Just as important, I need to let others own their feelings and not be quick in dismissing them.

This can be scary. We look into ourselves and ask, "Where did this feeling come from?" We need to identify it. Is it anger, insecurity, bitterness, resentment? By putting a label on it, we take away some of its power and control.

Finally, we need to figure out why we are feeling this right now and accept, or own, the feeling. This does not block us into corners, but instead sets us free.

I let myself own my feelings and set myself free for greater peacefulness.

Date / /

Today I Feel _____

_____

_____

_____

Lost Touch

Day 139

Disconnected sometimes describes our present relationship with our spouse. It's easy to become so obsessed with Lamaze classes, hospital tours and decorating the nursery that we lose touch with the person who cares for us so much.

Take a breather, put a halt to baby talk and return to the real world. Pretend for a day that we are not pregnant. Not talking about it forces us to concentrate on other topics. We could also take our spouse breakfast in bed or plan a favorite dinner. Our special friend needs us to pay attention to him because he misses us!

I take time today to "tickle the back" of the one I love and to spend time on other areas of my life.

Date / /

Today I Feel _____

Indecision

Day 140

Do we buy "generic" infant shirts? Or stick to the well-known brand that cost fifty cents more? Should we wear maternity hose or queen size regular? Minor decisions like these seem so difficult and we wonder why.

We are faced with so many choices now that the simpler ones seem burdensome. This overwhelming feeling about decision making is reflected in how we can't make the simplest of choices.

Overdependence on our partner may also occur. These are all symptoms of pregnancy stress and they will pass.

I take some quiet time to think about the decisions in my life, knowing that I can figure out what is right for me and my baby.

Date / /

Today I Feel _____

Resentment

Day 141

As much as we hate to admit it, we may feel some resentment about out pregnancy. We loved our life as it was, our marriage and the time to do what we wanted. Now, even before birth, we feel constraints. We can no longer sustain long car rides, stay up late at night, socialize all weekend or eat the food we love. We can only imagine what constraints will come with a baby.

How guilty we feel when we wish, just for a second, not to be pregnant. This is especially true if we had years of freedom. But then, when we think about our unborn child, our resentment is replaced with anticipation and joy.

Feeling resentment is natural, but my spiritual strength enables me to accept this and let go.

Date / /

Today I Feel _____

Ultrasound

Day 142

During our first trimester we may have had an ultrasound to determine the age of our baby or to tell if we are carrying twins. This sonogram probably did not mean much to us at the time. After all, who can make sense of shadows on photo paper? Now that we are further along and wondering how our baby is developing, some doctors routinely do another ultrasound. If we are worried about how our baby is developing, we may welcome another test. The fifteen minute procedure will relieve days of concern, thus reducing our stress.

Whenever possible, I choose to take any positive steps to be reassured that all is well within.

Date / /

Today I Feel

Simplify Life

Day 143

Short hair has finally won us over. We buy lunch at work every day. Paper plates are customary at dinner. Pizza is ordered twice a week. Does that sound familiar? The busier we become as our pregnancy progresses, the more we need to emphasize simplicity and shortcuts.

These are not examples of laziness but of our shifting priorities. We recognize that, as our responsibilities increase, something has to give.

A catnap is a better idea than feeling pressured to iron. Taking time for breakfast is more important than curling long hair. And getting to bed earlier is better than staying up making lunches.

Finding ways to economize time and energy is good preparation for parenthood.

Date / /

Today I Feel _____

_____

_____

_____

Hospitalization

Day 144

It is unfortunate if we have to go to the hospital while pregnant. We know we have good medical care, but being away from our family is upsetting for everyone.

Instead, let us find comfort in easing the distress of our other children. We can talk with them on the phone, let them visit or have Dad make video tapes.

The children can make cards for us or we could send pictures to them. Whatever we do, the children will sense that we love them. They will know we are maintaining our bond and not bitter about our developing baby.

*Getting outside myself by caring for others
helps me make the best of my situation.*

Date / /

Today I Feel _____

Comparison

Day 145

If we really want to get ourselves upset, all we have to do is start comparing our pregnancy to that of others. How much weight gained? What symptoms do you have? Inevitably we begin to question our physical status and lose self-confidence.

However, comparing is not fair to ourselves or anyone else. We are all individuals with specific needs and in different situations. No two pregnancies, two births or two babies are alike. We can learn from others' experiences, but we need to realize that all babies develop at their own pace, in their own time.

*Learning from others benefits me and my baby,
but expecting my experiences to be the same is not healthy.*

Date / /

Today I Feel

Willpower

Day 146

Being conscious about our actions can be difficult. With so much going on, it's very hard to keep track of what we eat and drink.

Visiting a friend, we find ourselves near a bowl of chips and dip. At work, a meeting starts with coffee and doughnuts. Three secretaries have candy dishes on their desks. And on Saturday, we only have time to grab some fast food while running errands.

Looking down at our stomachs, we say no one will notice a few extra pounds, but this philosophy will backfire. Too much weight gained will be difficult to lose afterwards. We need willpower to say no now and be glad later.

Do I want to be healthy later or not?

Date / /

Today I Feel _____

Stress

Day 147

You read a great article on C-sections and ask your husband to read it. He sets it aside and it stays there. You get on the scale at your doctor's and you've gained five pounds more than you thought. You share baby names with your family and they hate them all. Sound familiar?

Stress! Stress during pregnancy is the result of expectations not being met. We are already under pressure and adding the above can mean stress.

We need to recognize symptoms that show up as headaches, neck pain or backaches. Or less visible ones, such as depression, disorganization or anxiety.

I can find better ways to cope with stress in my life and decrease its debilitating presence.

Date / /

Today I Feel _____

_____

_____

_____

Trust

Day 148

Trust is such an important ingredient in raising a happy family and bringing a baby into the world. We must have trust in our partner, ourselves and our Higher Power. We must trust that we will never be alone in this experience.

How can we know that this trust really exists? Maybe by looking at the covenants in our lives. What covenant do we have with God? Ourselves? Our partner?

Covenants can be conscious or unconscious contracts, an understanding or mutual agreement. In our covenant, we trust those close to us.

I have a covenant of trust with my Higher Power, myself and my partner — in that order.

Date / /

Today I Feel _____

Superwoman

Day 149

Whether we admit it or not, there are a lot of added responsibilities now. This is the effect of adding the emotional and physical changes of pregnancy to our daily lives that were already full. We can be somewhat reassured knowing this is temporary.

The first step to reducing tension is to identify it. What pressures are we under each day? How can we lessen some of this?

We need to ask ourselves if we are trying to be superwomen. What pressures can we and others survive without?

I examine my responsibilities and discuss with family and co-workers how things could be made less stressful.

Date / /

Today I Feel _____

_____

_____

_____

Barriers

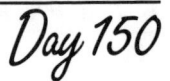

Day 150

As pregnancy progresses, we sometimes have difficulty accepting our condition. We wonder why we are not ecstatic. We want to have a baby, but the whole thing just doesn't feel positive all the time.

Identifying the barriers to enjoying our pregnancy is the first step. Do we have enough information? Do we feel the support and trust of others? Do we have a loving friend to share with? Barriers prevent us from feeling comfortable.

Working to understand why we don't feel comfortable with our pregnancy, we help ourselves come to terms with this life-changing experience. Our baby deserves a good start in life.

I will identify the barriers to happiness and start being proactive to create a peaceful pregnancy.

Date / /

Today I Feel _____

_____

_____

_____

Boundaries

Day 151

Somewhere along the way we may start to feel lost in all this baby stuff. We are surrounded by baby talk, pregnancy stories and medical facts. No one seems to remember the person we were before we got pregnant. As a result, we may feel as if we are losing our identity.

Without realizing it, we may be denying ourselves activities we enjoyed before. We need to set boundaries on how much this pregnancy will control our lives.

We need to rebalance our lives so that being pregnant is part of who we are, not the whole experience. Pregnancy and parenting itself take up our lives considerably, but balance still matters.

*I take time for me, giving myself what
I need to feel whole again.*

Date / /

Today I Feel _____

_____

_____

_____

Over-Reaction

Day 152

Not "crying over spilled milk" is difficult to do if we expect our lives to be perfect. This coupled with hormonal changes leads us to over-react to the most ridiculous things. Our worries about making wrong decisions and being perfect cause us to over-react.

We do not have to be the perfect pregnant woman, no matter how we define that. We may have a vision of how we expect ourselves to look or feel, but if we fall short or make some mistakes, this is okay. By forgiving ourselves, we will be able to move on, better prepared for the stresses of parenting.

Accepting myself and my limitations is the only way I will be at peace with myself.

Date / /

Today I Feel _____

Togetherness

Day 153

We are now not one, but two. Before long, there will be two persons here in this world, where there is so much love waiting to be shared. We will live together as two individuals, but as one team.

Life continues to go on around us as our baby grows each day. We find peace and beauty in the miracle of life as we live these quiet growing days together. Even now, with our baby still inside, we find our lives synchronized with him or her.

We realize this is why we are here: to love and experience life together with open hearts and minds. Our love has greatness and truth.

*Looking forward to sharing the life of my child,
I wait for our great love to begin.*

Date / /

Today I Feel _____

_____

_____

_____

Playtime

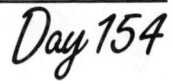

Day 154

When thinking of our baby growing up, we remember our own childhood. We may wish we were a child again, when things were so simple. Summer days seemed to last forever in backyards filled with baby frogs, white trilliums and a swing. The adults were always off doing "adult things" while we played and had fun.

The personal memories we hold within, whether good or bad, can be a foundation for building a life of memories for our baby. We will share with them the experiences that made us happy. At the same time, our children will open us up to new adventures.

I am glad that having a baby grants me the opportunity to reenter the world of play.

Date / /

Today I Feel _____

Emotions

Day 155

Many people dismiss our feelings during pregnancy as "normal" and due to hormones. Our emotional equilibrium is affected due to physical changes. Our entire body is altered by pregnancy.

We must remember that hormones are not the only thing influencing us. The attitudes of those around us can also affect us deeply. Our family, friends and co-workers need to try to understand what we are going through. Their positive attitudes help us develop an enthusiastic outlook.

When people are not positive toward my pregnancy, I communicate how I feel. I can't control their attitudes, but I can tell them if they continue, they will alienate me.

Date / /

Today I Feel _____

Memory

Day 156

Our grandmothers have probably played an important part in our lives. If we are lucky, they still may be living to share this baby with us. If they have died, we will share favorite grandmother stories with our children.

For each of us, the special times are different. Some grandmothers are known for wonderful recipes that can be passed down. Others are remembered for birthday baskets filled with lotions, soaps and candies.

Memories are God's gift to us for our own older days. We will soon be creating many new memories for both ourselves and our own children.

Those who are close and dear to me are remembered as I share memories with my own child.

Date / /

Today I Feel _____

_____

_____

_____

Anticipation

Day 157

Why do we do this to ourselves? We fret about future events that may or may not take place or fears that may have to be faced. Being anxious we only create stress for ourselves, our baby and those around us. We develop a kind of stage fright, with our energies focused on the future instead of the present. The more we look into the future, the higher the level of anxiety we bring upon ourselves. We have no control over the future, only of present events. We can only control the future when it becomes our present.

I stay in touch with how I focus my energy to cope with everyday demands and reduce anxiety about the future.

Date / /

Today I Feel _____

Faith

Day 158

For many people, faith is trust that life will unfold according to the plan of a Higher Power. Is this how we feel about faith during pregnancy?

We are now faced with many new concerns and worries, but in faith we find peace. A gift given to comfort us, faith is the way we let go of our worries and give them over to God. The miracle of our baby's healthy development is in His hands.

Faith shelters us from worry that can drain us of energy. It gives us the promise of hope and happiness. Faith offers peace of mind and a joyful heart.

I have faith and surrender my worries to my Higher Power, freeing myself of their shadow.

Date / /

Today I Feel _____

_____

_____

_____

Attachment

Day 159

What level of attachment do we feel toward our unborn child? There's no right or wrong sense of attachment we're supposed to feel at any specific time. Every expectant mother's process of bonding differs.

For some of us it may have started with the idea of getting pregnant. Once pregnant, we imagined what the baby would look like and felt a closeness begin. For others, fetal movement or hearing the heartbeat generates a sense of closeness. Or attachment may begin during birth, or afterwards when we actually see our child.

In its own right time, the experience of bonding occurs between me and my child.

Date / /

Today I Feel _____

Pediatric Care

Day 160

One responsibility we have is to arrange for postnatal care of our baby. We will want to select a pediatrician who has a good reputation and can provide the level of care we want.

We should make an office visit, check out the facility and meet the staff. Bringing a list of questions helps us remember our concerns. What are their hours? Is someone available on call? What is the payment arrangement?

The health care of our children during their growing years is one of our primary concerns. We must be certain that we can depend on health professionals to give good care to our children.

I take the time to make a careful decision about my child's health care.

Date / /

Today I Feel

Tiredness

Day 161

There will be no escaping fatigue during pregnancy. It is a common condition as well as a side effect especially granted to those who try to be superwomen.

We can help ourselves to more peacefulness by prioritizing our responsibilities daily. It's okay to do the minimum some days. We must not feel guilty when we look at unwashed dishes, bulging laundry piles or an unbalanced checkbook. Housework can wait. What can't wait is the nap we desperately need, the help our other children need with homework, cuddling with our husbands or a relaxing bubble bath.

Being tired means being miserable and skews my perspective of my world, so I spend my energy carefully.

Date / /

Today I Feel _____

Understanding

Day 162

"You'll understand someday when you have children of your own." Since we are now having our own, we will soon be able to understand this statement. No longer will we be kept out of this exclusive club!

Another saying we were subjected to was "You can only understand if you carry a baby for nine months." That is something that we can already relate to. We feel a depth of love we never before thought possible. Once our child is born, we will further understand these statements. Will we manage not to pass on such an exclusive attitude to our own children?

Certain aspects of life have more meaning when we become pregnant and raise a child.

Date / /

Today I Feel

Public Property

Day 163

As we walk into the elevator, a man asks, "When are you due?" Later a waiter asks, "You aren't drinking, are you?" A co-worker rubs our stomach and a clerk at the market stares us up and down.

These are the daily experiences of expectant women. We become public property! At first we like it, but as months pass, we get tired of it. We should remind ourselves that later, our babies will receive much more attention. People will want to hold them, strangers will touch them and friends will give advice. How do we plan on dealing with this? Can we communicate our needs to friends and accept the rest graciously?

I try to remain positive toward those around me, seeing their attention as love.

Date / /

Today I Feel

Accidents

Day 164

As pregnancy progresses, our clumsiness increases. We become more off balance due to bodily changes, which can cause accidents and injury.

How can we possibly remember every time to be careful? The answer is quite simple: out of necessity for our well being and that of our babies.

All it takes is a split second to miss that bottom step or fall as we're hanging a picture or putting up curtain rods. If we're not careful, we could injure ourselves and even affect the development of the baby. Why take unnecessary risks?

I try to be more patient now and use more common sense in accomplishing things.

Date / /

Today I Feel

Independence

Day 165

What will our primary goals be after we have our baby? On the top of our list will be nurturing the baby through developmental stages. What we really will be doing is preparing them to handle life on their own. They will need to depend on themselves eventually, not us.

This is not sad, but a healthy, happy process. We will experience much joy as we watch our newborns, infants, children and then adolescents spread their wings. Our guidance will prepare them for an autonomous life separate from us. In spirit, though, we will always be connected.

As my pregnancy progresses, I think about my goals as a parent.

Date / /

Today I Feel _____

Bed Rest

Day 166

We can anticipate many things during pregnancy, but may be taken by surprise if we are told to stay in bed to avoid premature labor. Imposed rest may seem wonderful at first, but concern for the baby can be stressful. Because we may feel guilty relying on others, communication with our family is crucial. We are all working toward a shared goal: a healthy baby. Another difficult feeling will be loneliness, as we spend so much time in bed alone. It may feel uncomfortable, but as time passes, we become more peaceful about this situation. We know that the healthy development of our baby is most important.

While bed-bound, I keep a routine, try to occupy myself and depend on others and my Higher Power.

Date / /

Today I Feel _____

Seeking Peace

Day 167

Feeling pulled in every direction can be stressful, even without pregnancy. We need to remind ourselves now that it's okay to depend on others to help us find peace on our daily journey. There's no way we can take care of everything around us. Family members, friends and support groups are there for us, especially when we feel that everything is just too much to handle.

When we get to the breaking point, we need to let go and let God guide us. Soon our lives will return to a feeling of balance and inner peace.

I give over my stressed-out life to my Higher Power, knowing this is the source of my peacefulness.

Date / /

Today I Feel _____

Showers

Day 168

Traditional baby showers, father showers, office and work showers, couple showers, second baby showers, adoption showers and family showers seem to be given in abundance these days. Before, as observers, we may have wondered what all the fuss was about. Now we look forward to our own baby shower because it has a new meaning for us. It seems much more than just a party to take up an afternoon.

We will enjoy the gifts and food, but more important is the rite of passage that this represents. We will be surrounded by those closest to us to share our happiness and celebrate the miracle of new life.

Perspective and opinions about things change as I enter into my new world.

Date / /

Today I Feel _____

_____

_____

_____

Judging

Day 169

"Do you think she's pregnant or just putting on weight?" We may have heard people asking each other this, especially if we are older than the average pregnant woman. Until our third trimester, we may experience some stares and questions.

Judging, criticizing and not accepting are all signs of insecurity. People tend to feel threatened by differences or uncommon situations. With the increasing number of older moms, this is changing and those who find it unusual are increasingly in the minority!

> *I feel compassionate toward those who stare because they are the ones with a problem.*

Date / /

Today I Feel _____

New Center

Day 170

Soon there will be a new center to our world: the life of our newborn! We will have the joy of watching a new person develop, change and grow. Our unknown entity will no longer be the mystery it is now. A personality will emerge that we will be able to witness from an innocent little person who blossoms into a child and then an adult. Our lives will never be the same. At first our equilibrium will seem way off, but then it will feel the most balanced ever! The center of our lives becomes our baby, and that is the way it has to be until our new life becomes independent and can survive on its own.

I take the responsibility of giving this new life center the attention and care it needs.

Date / /

Today I Feel _____

Calling

Day 171

It is a very great calling to be asked to love another human being, especially a child. We have committed ourselves to the development of another human being. We have chosen to make sacrifice and responsibility part of our daily lives.

We will be looking for ways to improve and guide our baby's life. We will be increasing the quality of our lives and equipping our child with skills, self-esteem and confidence.

We are called to be the best role model we can be for our developing child. This commitment is for the long haul, as we guide this new person in life.

*I respond to the call with all the love
and tenderness that is in me.*

Date / /

Today I Feel ___

War Stories

Day 172

For years, we may have heard "war stories" from the men in our families. They spend hours reminiscing about their experiences, recounting their courage and ability to survive.

Women do the same thing with stories about labor and delivery. Grandmothers, aunts and sisters sit around during family reunions retelling how long they were in labor, how poor the medical care was or how uncaring the nurses.

What stories will we have to tell? Sharing with other women is wonderful, but we shouldn't listen too closely. After all, just as with war stories, these tend to have a certain embellishment.

*Family stories are a great tradition and
I savor the connection and sharing.*

Date / /

Today I Feel _____

Isolation

Day 173

Those who are married or living with partners are lucky to have someone to give support when needed. But we who are having our babies as single parents are much more challenged. This situation can cause isolation, making us feel alone, irritable and impatient. At these times we need to depend on our network of friends and family. Little breaks for a walk, grocery shopping or church allow us much relief.

We also need to depend on our Higher Power for guidance. From this source we receive strength to endure the exhausting times and energy to replace burnout.

As a single parent, I feel down at times, but I begin now to depend on my friends, family and Higher Power.

Date / /

Today I Feel _____

The Climb

Day 174

We can think of life as a big mountain that we have chosen to climb together. We will encounter challenges, such as having a child, but certain concepts help us through. First, we must work to define our goals. We want to get somewhere together and we need to share our dreams and then plan for them.

Second, we must realize that there will be setbacks. One may stumble, but the other will be there to help.

As we continue, we must also be in touch with our spiritual side and share this as a family. Our Higher Power is the strength for our continued climb.

Thinking of life as a climb together creates a team spirit necessary for reaching our family goals.

Date / /

Today I Feel _____

Dreams

Day 175

Our days remain very busy. We take care of our homes and family matters, try to keep up with our work and maintain some kind of social life. During this rigorous time, we may not be consciously thinking about problems; we just have so many externals to be concerned with.

But in our dreams these unsettling concerns may appear. Dreams can be very symbolic and very vivid. During a time when our emotions are very intense, dreams are very healing, although disturbing. Remember, even when dreams are frightening, every night has a sunrise.

My dreams are not predictions of what will happen, but an outlet for anxieties. If I have a dream that bothers me, I share it with someone I trust.

Date / /

Today I Feel _____

Sequencing

Day 176

"Sequencing" is a form of compromise for women who want both a career and children. The concept is not new in practice, but it is now more clearly defined, talked about and accepted. It is a way for us to find balance and satisfaction in our lives.

The first phase of sequencing is working before we have children. We save money, develop job skills and get to know our partners.

The second phase is when we have our families and work fewer hours at a job. We raise our children and work part-time. Phase three follows when we reenter the work force full time.

I discuss my work plans with my partner and consider sequencing.

Date / /

Today I Feel _____

Strength

Day 177

Some days we feel extremely strong, glowing with vitality. Other days, we can barely roll out of bed, feeling weak and incapable. We know deep in our hearts that our strength will return, but we also know we have some struggles ahead.

The closer in spirit we are to our Higher Power, the more peace of mind we will find. When trying to get our day started, we need to let go and trust fully. God will guide us through the day and give us patience, especially with the simple things in life. Parenting is a particularly good area in life to practice letting go, for no one can do it alone, either before or after birth.

Be near to me, God, and watch over me and my family throughout this day.

Date   /   /

Today I Feel _____

_____

_____

_____

Working

Day 178

All along, we have said that we will return to work after the baby comes. After all, we worked hard to get where we are in our careers. We need the income to continue living the way we do. Or we may need the income just to survive and have no choice.

Whatever our situation, we now may be questioning this decision. Our jobs may seem less significant compared to a child. We may worry about the quality of child care. Or we may realize how much we're looking forward to being at home for the first time in years.

We naturally wonder about our work plans as the reality of a baby sinks in.

I evaluate my work situation and make whatever decision is right for my family.

Date / /

Today I Feel

T.L.C.

Day 179

Are we feeling in the dumps because we have not slept through the night in weeks? Are we feeling sick with the stress of everything we're dealing with? We need to make sure we take care of ourselves no matter how busy we get.

We can do many things to improve our disposition: take a bubble bath, read a novel, take a long nap or talk to a close friend. We all have unique ways of relaxing and enjoying ourselves. We'd better do these things now because once the baby comes, we'll have little free time. Giving ourselves some tender, loving care every day helps any situation we are in.

Starting today, I take measures to counter the stress in my life.

Date / /

Today I Feel

Daydreams

Day 180

Images may repeat themselves in our minds during the strangest times of the day, creating fearful scenes of harm for our future child. Bizarre fantasies can haunt us and we wonder why. We are lovingly looking forward to parenting. How can we imagine danger?

These daydreams may be offering us a learning tool for parenting. We are concerned about the safety of our baby or lack confidence in ourselves as parents. These daydreams indicate our inner concerns. We can take time to analyze them, discuss our fears and regain our peaceful pregnancy.

I acknowledge my fearful fantasies, but then disempower them with positivism.

Date / /

Today I Feel _____

Realistic Expectations

Day 181

Do we really know what is in store for us after the birth? Do we have this fantasy of a happy family where Daddy returns home from work to a smiling baby, a well-rested Mom and dinner on the table? Just what do we expect?

We need to ask ourselves how we define parenting. If we are uncertain about this, now is an excellent time to talk with other parents. We could spend time with an infant or visit a nursery. The more we know what to expect, the better we will be able to cope with the demands and to help each other out in a confident manner.

I need to think realistically about the demands of parenthood, which will constantly change for years to come.

Date / /

Today I Feel

Old Tapes

Day 182

Things could not be better for us. We feel wonderful and our lives are going great. Our life seems under control and we bask in the joy of our pregnancy.

Then we run into an old girlfriend, someone we grew up with but had lost track of. We did everything together before we had a major falling out. We had planned to live on the same street when we grew up and have our children grow up together. Seeing her now, we feel uncomfortable and a little out of control.

We both try to find the right words to exchange, trying to regain contact out of separate worlds that have changed drastically.

> *As difficult as it is, I let go of the past and erase the old tapes that replay in my mind.*

Date / /

Today I Feel _____

Openness

Day 183

Plans for pregnancy, birth and postpartum may already be established in our minds. We know exactly how we want things to progress, methods we will use and what kind of parents we will be. Are we sure this is the best approach? Could we be setting ourselves up for disappointments?

These are such complicated experiences that they rarely go the way women think they will. Instead of being set in our ideas, why not try to be flexible? We need to be open to any possibility. Pregnancy is a process that presents us with many surprises. Our expectations may change as pregnancy progresses.

I need to take one day at a time and remain open to anything.

Date / /

Today I Feel

Past Memories

Day 184

While we are pregnant, good and bad memories of our childhoods can be stirred up. Incidents come to mind that we have not thought of in years. Although it feels good to reminisce about the happy experiences, others can bring pain.

Maybe this is a good time to examine some of that pain. Where does it come from? Why does it still exist? And what can we do to eliminate it? Having a baby is a new beginning for us, as well as for the other members of our family. Often a new baby can be the catalyst to break down family bitterness and bring forgiveness and love.

Let my baby and our happiness be a means of healing my family and bringing us together in love.

Date / /

Today I Feel _____

Low-Risk

Day 185

Becoming a mother for the first time can be very scary. We spend months preparing as the excitement builds. Until now, we may have had a low-risk pregnancy without complications. However, this label can change at any point.

Many reasons can lead to a high-risk situation. Most likely, however, it is nothing that we did or didn't do. Fetal distress, breech position or overdue pregnancy can happen to any expectant mother for any reason. This may lead to inducement, medication or even a Cesarean section. Remember that having a healthy baby should remain our objective.

I am thankful for every day my pregnancy is considered low-risk.

Date / /

Today I Feel

Need

Day 186

Remember when the family dinner lasted for hours? Remember when we slept in until ten on Saturday mornings? Our needs are beginning to change, such as how we spend our time and what is important to us.

The family's need for us also is changing. Our other children may need us a lot more until they feel less threatened by the new baby. Our husband's need for us may vacillate or increase as the due date approaches.

After the baby comes, it may seem as if everyone needs us all the time. As the family becomes used to the new circumstances, their needs will decrease.

*I pray I will have the energy and patience to
meet the needs of those around me —
with a little left over for myself.*

Date / /

Today I Feel _____

Rotten

Day 187

"Rotten" may very well be the word to describe how we've been feeling the last couple of weeks. Everything is going fine, we're both healthy, but overall we just feel plain old rotten. We must remind ourselves that this is only a temporary state and that soon we will resume our normal energy level, physical agility and interest in sex.

If we find this turning into real depression, feeling as if there is no hope of things improving, we need to get some help. By sharing these feelings with someone we trust, we gain our sense of balance again. Confronting negative emotions is the way to diffuse them.

If I feel constantly rotten, talking helps restore my peaceful pregnancy.

Date / /

Today I Feel _____

Surrender

Day 188

For the rest of our lives we will be responsible for another human being. The degree of care will change, but not the bond. We will end up surrendering a lot of ourselves to this new person as required of us as parents.

Every aspect of our lives will be changed. We rejoice in knowing that ahead of us lie challenge, work, joy, happiness and growth. Surrendering ourselves to another human being is what life is all about. Caring leads to maturation and deeper understanding. Instead of seeing our freedom as being taken away, we can think of parenting as giving us more.

The more I give of myself, the more I learn about my values and beliefs.

Date / /

Today I Feel

Third Trimester

Being Heard

Day 189

At the end of the day, we may be feeling frustrated but can't figure out why. It may be because all day we never felt heard. At work, the manager kept bothering us. At lunch, acquaintances kept interrupting our conversation with a friend. And later, our doctor talked on and on. In all these instances, no one asked us how we felt.

We need to know that the significant people in our lives — family, friends, co-workers and doctor — are listening to us and that we are being heard. Especially now it is important for us to feel that our needs matter to others and that we have their support.

> *I communicate my needs to others and let them see how I need their support.*

Date / /

Today I Feel _____

Nourishment

Day 190

The pace of physical changes to our baby during the last trimester is phenomenal. Even though the body has fully formed, nails grow, hair appears, features sharpen, skin becomes smooth, eyelashes develop and fatty plumpness is added. These are the final touches preparing for the upcoming main event!

We need to read about and discuss these changes with others to have a better understanding of how we affect the development. This growth compares with the changes our babies will experience during their first year of life. These changes are truly miraculous.

Just as imperative as prenatal care is the nurturing I give my baby after birth and throughout her life.

Date / /

Today I Feel _____

Loving Touch

Day 191

Affection is one of the most important ingredients in a good marriage. If you do not believe it, try this experiment. Next time you feel upset about anything, ask your husband or child for some hugs. After a few minutes, see how you feel. It's almost guaranteed that you will feel a much stronger sense of personal worth, security and love.

Affectionate touching eases many strains we may suffer. It communicates that the person is special and loved, and it strengthens family ties.

> *The sense of touch is a warm, secure way*
> *of showing others I love them, and is*
> *especially good for me and my baby.*

Date   /   /

Today I Feel _____

Love

Day 192

"Will I love my baby from the first moment?" For months we have imagined that special moment when our baby is handed to us for the first time. Yet doubt lurks in our hearts because we wonder how we will feel. Will we be euphoric? Or will our baby seem like a complete stranger making us feel full of guilt?

Thinking about this now helps us avoid certain expectations. We can't know how we will feel. We could be drugged up from a Cesarean or we could be so drained from labor we just sleep until the next day. This process of bonding, however, is something that takes place over a long period of time, with many years ahead.

Love takes time to develop, but with patience
I will adore my new child.

Date   /   /

Today I Feel

One At A Time

Day 193

We know deep down from our own experiences that everything passes in due time. Unfortunately we don't always have the luxury of knowing how long. With labor, at least we know there has to be a finite ending, and in this we can find comfort.

Labor is a temporary state like any other experience. We know an average labor lasts eight to twelve hours. By focusing on its transitory state and taking one contraction at a time, we will feel more at ease. We know, too, that in coping with labor we will become strengthened. With all our physical and emotional pain, a new awareness will be born.

I know I have strength and wisdom from past experiences to help me endure labor.

Date / /

Today I Feel

Falling Apart

Day 194

Some days we feel as if we are falling apart at the seams. We can't figure out where these days come from, how they develop or why they get so intense. But they do exist and they seem to last forever. Everything we do is wrong and everything we try is met with an obstruction to our goals. Obviously we're out of sync with the whole universe.

What is a woman in our condition to do with a day like this? We can share such a day with a close friend. She will listen, make us laugh and point out how funny life is. Such sharing with friends lifts our spirits and helps us retain our peacefulness.

Close friends and my Higher Power are what redeem days when my life falls apart.

Date / /

Today I Feel _____

Bonding

Day 195

We may already feel deep love for our baby. This is demonstrated in how we reach down and touch our stomach or rub it rhythmically while lying down. This affection is important and wonderful. Our baby is with us twenty-four hours a day, going through phenomenal changes, just as we are.

This beginning bonding is healthy and good to express. Once our baby is born, our love will feel even more natural, an extension of the affection we have already been experiencing. For now, we bond with what we imagine our baby to be like inside and what the future holds.

Today I take extra time to be quiet with my baby, listening to his movements and feeling close.

Date / /

Today I Feel _____

Extended Family

Day 196

In the past, many family members lived under one roof. Today grandparents, brothers and sisters usually live elsewhere, often far away. But we can still benefit from the knowledge and support they have to offer during visits or by phone.

Each family has people who inspire and motivate. These people teach us about life and motherhood. They can lend a hand when we need it, give us emotional support and share their experiences. This "extended family" will be wonderful for our baby, too. He or she will learn a lot from a different set of arms.

My baby and I are fortunate to have family members to inspire and love us.

Date / /

Today I Feel _____

Labor Pain

Day 197

Fear of labor is natural and common. Although we may have experienced some physical discomfort in the past, labor is different and unknown. We ask, "Can I deal with the pain? Will I have the help I need? What does a contraction feel like?"

Although we can't control or cancel our labor, we can prepare ourselves. Confronting our fear is a beginning. Childbirth classes, exercise and good nutrition are a good start, but we also may need extra help with pain control. Our doctor can tell us what medication is available. We want what is best for our baby, but also best for ourselves. Labor is not meant to be an enemy, but a friend helping our bodies deliver our baby.

Practicing a positive, accepting attitude helps me through the birthing process, "one contraction at a time."

Date / /

Today I Feel

Growth

Day 198

The growth and development of a person takes a long time and is filled with many experiences. We can be very impatient with ourselves and our family, especially now.

Even as supportive as he is, our husband still may not realize the strains of our pregnancy. Instead of trying to make changes, we can accept him, knowing he will change when he is ready.

After months of pregnancy, we see many changes within ourselves. We now also want to see changes in those we love, to feel the security of being on the same wavelength. But people change when it's right for them.

*I see many changes in myself, but I try
not to expect this from others.*

Date / /

Today I Feel _____

_____

_____

_____

Working

Day 199

Soon we may be faced with combining mothering and working. Many demands will be placed on us as we try to give our all to both. We may have considered working part-time or out of our home, but for some of us these are not options. We worry about how we will cope after the birth. "What if the babysitter gets sick? What if there isn't enough money? What if the baby has special needs? What if I can't handle the stress?"

What good does it do to worry about things that may not happen? We can't predict the future. There are ways to prepare, but it does not help to worry over possibilities.

I set reasonable expectations for the present and try not to second-guess the future.

Date / /

Today I Feel _____

Thankfulness

Day 200

Have we taken time today to reflect on the good aspects of our lives? Our health, homes, loved ones, food or job? Have we expressed thankfulness to our Higher Power, our spouses or ourselves for the simple pleasures we are privileged to experience? Such things can be a good night's rest, a warm cup of tea, a flutter in our womb or unswollen ankles.

We are all too quick to dwell on the trials in our lives, self-pitying and sulking when life does not go our way. During these times we can find comfort in the simple pleasures we do have. When we encounter hardship, we have more peace of mind if we center on the good in our lives.

I work on being at peace with myself, in harmony with the wonder of birth.

Date / /

Today I Feel _____

The Silence

Day 201

As we listen to the silence, we dream wonderful visions of our child. We see the time ahead as we daily experience our child's development. We think of all the things our child will learn to do, all the beautiful times we will share. We know the future holds many things, great joy and perhaps great sorrow. Being granted the privilege of parenthood will initiate us into a complex world of love, struggle, worry and joy.

Spending time alone by ourselves during pregnancy is a good way to become more comfortable with the idea of parenting. We are becoming something we have never been before and it takes some getting used to.

*Silence offers me a valuable space where
I find strength, comfort and peace.*

Date / /

Today I Feel _____

Nearness

Day 202

Thoughts and visions of our baby crowd our minds right now. Pictures of holding them, having them near us and rocking them are foremost in our thoughts. Soon the infant we have imagined for so long will become real.

Right now there is no division between us. We are one and will continue to be so for a short time longer. Each day we cherish this time because it will be gone before we know it.

Our mental preoccupation is preparing us for the actual nearness of our baby. We know that by having our baby, we will leave this world better, filled with more laughter and love.

*I find much comfort by imagining
my baby near me.*

Date / /

Today I Feel _____

Anxiety

Day 203

Life may seem to be going smoothly for us. We go about our normal routine, running errands, going to work or talking on the phone. Then when we least expect it, we feel a clutch of alarm. We feel helpless, scared and nervous. "Oh, my God, what am I doing? Am I really having a baby?"

Even though we're in our last months, we may still experience this. In time it passes and then we try to analyze it. Distressing emotions are normal during pregnancy. Love, security and joy can't be felt all forty weeks. Occasional anxiety is part of going beyond ourselves and into changing times of growth.

I find comfort in knowing that as I travel through my anxiety, I begin to lose it.

Date / /

Today I Feel _____

Parents

Day 204

In the eyes of children, parents can be the most beautiful creatures God has created. When the whole world comes crashing down on them, we bring comfort and help them learn independence. Through the years the trust between us will grow as they learn we will always be there for them with love and guidance.

Our child will be lucky because many children in the world don't have loving parents. These children do not have loving arms to turn to that help them see that life is a gift. As we begin as parents, we should feel good about our loving intentions.

I have so much to give my child through her growing years that I look forward to welcoming her into the world.

Date / /

Today I Feel _____

Celebration

Day 205

We will soon be celebrating a new beginning! With the birth of our baby, family and friends will gather to celebrate. This birth means that the family tree will continue and bring future generations. A sense of healthy content, promise and hope arises.

As expectant mothers, we have been celebrating in our hearts all along. The actual birth will only be an external manifestation of what we've been feeling daily for months. A birth is a wonderful thing for families, bringing together alienated relatives and healing wounds.

I revel in my daily inner celebration that marks the coming birth of my child.

Date / /

Today I Feel _____

_____

_____

_____

Quiet

Day 206

Sometimes when the day is over and darkness comes to the sky, a great sense of peace settles over us. We can try to find its source by looking at the people around us, watching and listening. We can go into the baby's room and touch the crib or little T-shirts.

We sit in the rocking chair and stare at the silver moon through the window. As we close our eyes, a great quiet comes over us as we sense the center of this peace. We did not need to search far. As we rock, we realize all we needed to do was reach down and touch our expanding abdomen.

The quiet, warmth and movements are peaceful gifts for me to experience in joyful waiting.

Date / /

Today I Feel _____

Second Chance

Day 207

Childhood for some of us was very hard, filled with fear, unhappiness, abuse and little love. We have learned to put it in the past and move on. However, now that we're becoming parents, our confidence in raising a child differently may be waning. Maybe if we take a positive, different approach, we will feel more secure.

We can think of our baby as a second chance for us. We won't be living our lives through our children, but setting our hearts to make life better for them. This act of love will create special times for our family. We can find comfort in knowing that our efforts will heal our past and create happy memories for our child.

I can't change my childhood, but now I have a second chance with my own child.

Date / /

Today I Feel _____

Danger

Day 208

Danger may become a component of our pregnancy. Perhaps physical conditions bring on complications or we live in a dangerous environment. Each of us knows our own personal dangers and how they affect us.

We know the power that danger can have over us and our lives, how we can be manipulated and changed. The only way to escape the danger in our lives is to avoid it or get away from it. If this is not possible, then we must stand steadfast, trust in our Higher Power and confront the danger head on.

*I must take action against any danger in my life,
to find freedom and safety for myself
and my unborn child.*

Date / /

Today I Feel _____

Twelve Steps

Day 209

Although many of us may have been working on the Twelve Steps or other self-help programs before our pregnancy, they were always tied to some disorder. We must remember that now they are a way of life, not just tools for crises. There are emotional struggles throughout pregnancy. With the aid of self-help programs, friends and our Higher Power, we have the courage for this unfamiliar territory. We appreciate the uniqueness of this learning situation and its unlimited possibilities. By recognizing and accepting, we begin to feel free from our fears.

I continue living one day at a time and make use of resources such as the Twelve Steps.

Date / /

Today I Feel

Education

Day 210

At the beginning of our pregnancy we were motivated to find out all about this experience. We wanted to know what was going to happen to our bodies for the next nine months.

Now we need to educate ourselves for labor and delivery. The more we know and understand, the more our fears will subside. We need to know about effacement, dilation, early labor signs, active labor, transition, pushing positions and delivery. With each, there are different physical and emotional responses, coping techniques, and recommendations for our support people.

*I continue to maintain my self-care attitude because
I am valuable and deserve this attention.*

Date / /

Today I Feel

Outside The Womb

Day 211

For forty weeks we carry a life within our womb, feeling it move and planning for its arrival. Very soon we will be able to see, smell, touch and hold our own "flesh and blood." This person will need a lot of love once life begins. Our new relationship will begin developing.

Now a whole new set of concerns will replace the ones we had throughout pregnancy. No matter how we try to prepare ourselves, unknown situations will arise, just as they have the last few months. The strength we gain in pregnancy will help us learn all about parenting.

I try not to obsess about how things may be after the baby arrives, but do what I can to prepare and enjoy what is happening now.

Date / /

Today I Feel _____

Appearance

Day 212

At this point, we may be looking at ourselves thinking, "So huge!" Our maternity clothes don't look as cute. We've added a "waddle" to our walk and stretch marks have appeared all over our bodies. Friends say how wonderful we look, but that doesn't help. On days like this, we must remind ourselves that the most important thing is our health and the health of our baby. This stage is only temporary and we will get the chance to trim down after the baby comes. Looking at it from another perspective, our large size is a gorgeous statement of life.

I remind myself that this condition is temporary and once I have the baby, I can concentrate on getting back "in shape."

Date / /

Today I Feel _____

Premature

Day 213

Despite our efforts and our doctor's care, we still could go into labor early. This thought plagues every expectant mother.

We need to know if we are at risk and what the signs are. Knowing procedures in case of premature labor also helps.

Information is power and helps us feel more in control. We find further comfort in knowing medical advances now exist to control early labor. Many hospitals also have excellent neonatal units.

Most importantly, we need to remind ourselves of the presence of our Higher Power for guidance and strength.

If labor begins early, I trust my Higher Power, my doctor and my own inner strength to see us through.

Date / /

Today I Feel _____

Unknown

Day 214

The unknown can be scary: a new job, leaving our spouse, attending a new class or having a baby. We can alleviate some trepidation by preparing ourselves.

One way to be ready for labor is to tour the birthing facility at the hospital. Seeing the actual delivery room, touring the nursery and meeting the staff increase our confidence. This proactive step prevents anxiety as we greet the unknown instead of waiting for it to greet us. Another important way to help ourselves is by continuing to trust in our Higher Power and a dependable coach.

I have the power to make things happen that will help me face impending change.

Date / /

Today I Feel

Time Urgency

Day 215

Forty long weeks of gestation and yet there still seems to be too much to do. A sense of "time urgency" may be what we have been feeling lately. We do everything in a hurried fashion, not slow and concentrated as we did before.

Our lifestyles have been altered. No longer can we depend on preplanning, routines and organized activities. These are completely dependent on how we feel at the time. If we are too exhausted, we postpone them until we feel better. Then, when we have energy, we have a million things to do . . . or so it seems! At this point, we have a strong sense that we have lost a certain control over our time.

When I feel I can't catch my breath, I put my feet up and force myself to relax.

Date / /

Today I Feel _____

Awakening

Day 216

All of a sudden we wake up one morning and realize, as if for the first time, that very soon we will become parents. Sure, we have been thinking about it for a long time, but now it feels different, more real.

What we are feeling is an awakening. For the last few months we have been in the process of "becoming," and now the time is coming to take on the responsibility of parenting. The process of becoming is almost over.

Our pregnancy has enabled us to experience new joy and challenge. We will never be able to return to the people we were before. We have stretched to new horizons.

I treasure this "awakening" as a special gift
I am knowing for the first time.

Date   /   /

Today I Feel _____

_____

_____

_____

Weight Gain

Day 217

At the beginning of our pregnancy, we had a goal for weight gain. But as months passed, we may have gained more each month than we had anticipated. Now we get on the scale and are a bit shocked.

Our doctor can oversee our nutritional habits and tell us what weight gain is healthy. The issue of weight gain is less stressed than years ago. Now, if we are eating healthy foods and getting some exercise, we shouldn't obsess about weight. We must be gentle with ourselves. After all, some weight must be gained to support a healthy developing baby, which is our main objective. Right?

I follow the advice of my doctor on weight, but try not to fall into the trap of weight obsession.

Date   /   /

Today I Feel _____

_____

_____

_____

Disability

Day 218

All of us are human creatures trying to make our way through life. When we were not pregnant, we had energy we could depend on. Now, in the later stages of pregnancy or "far along," we may feel disabled in some ways.

Being physically challenged for the first time can be scary and frustrating. No longer do we climb the stairs at work, but take the nearest elevator instead. No longer can we take long hikes around the park, but feel lucky just to get that far. No longer can we shop and feel like one of the crowd.

This experience humbles me and forces me to become more compassionate toward those who are truly disabled.

Date / /

Today I Feel

Gift

Day 219

Feelings about life's circumstances can be confusing and even illogical. For instance, when we experience a rough time, we think we deserve it. We become martyrs and develop the "poor me" syndrome. Can we honestly say we do the same when good happens? Of course not. Instead, we think we don't deserve it or it was a fluke. We still feel inadequate and defeated.

Beginning today we can turn this around by praising ourselves for the good we have allowed to come into our lives. The life within us is a special gift our Higher Power has bestowed on us — a gift of love for years to come.

*Having a baby is a gift, a real dream come true and
I will not rob myself of its special pleasure.*

Date / /

Today I Feel _____

_____

_____

_____

Relentless Giving

Day 220

Have we seriously thought about "giving"? What role does it play in our lives? Do we value this characteristic in others? Would we define ourselves as generous?

We need to think about giving now because once the baby comes, we will have to give relentlessly of our time, energy, finances and love. It will be a never-ending experience of giving that can be quite draining. It will literally encompass all of us, something we have never known before. An innocent, helpless baby will be totally dependent on us.

> ***Before the baby arrives, I practice giving with family and friends.***

Date / /

Today I Feel _____

Separation

Day 221

As our pregnancy progresses, we seem to be making decisions that separate us from our partner. We re-evaluate our current lifestyle, environment and activities. We may decide that certain behaviors are not healthy for us or our baby.

We may even feel that we need to consider leaving our partner if he refuses to change, particularly if he is addicted or violent. Too much is at risk now to continue with things the way they have been. We do not have to do anything that we are not emotionally ready for, but we will know instinctively if this is the right move.

Any relationship must be right and healthy for me, my baby and our future.

Date / /

Today I Feel _____

Gratitude

Day 222

Tonight we stretch out our arms and ask for direction during the remaining weeks of pregnancy. We ask for hope to remain positive and to reduce stress. We thank our Higher Power for taking us this far in our journey and share our gratitude with others.

Gratitude is such a wonderful tool. It strengthens us and makes us feel good about our present state of mind. When we feel grateful, we are recognizing gifts we have been given in our lives. During these last few months we have struggled, but we have been strengthened as we welcome a new person into our lives.

Feeling grateful for the blessings of my life,
such as my pregnancy, fulfills my
spirit and strengthens my days.

Date / /

Today I Feel _____

New Life Adventure

Day 223

After all of our effort during our pregnancy, we have life's greatest adventure ahead of us. Birth is not the main event, even though we have been focusing on it for so long. Birth is merely a doorway to our new life as parents.

Overwhelmed may be the best word to describe the thought of this! But, taking one day at a time, little by little, is the way to maintain serenity. With this philosophy we experience a growing sense of confidence with our new status. We will feel more comfortable with the new responsibilities of being a mother.

So many gifts await me as I become this new person, a mother.

Date / /

Today I Feel _____

Fact

Day 224

"What if the baby is retarded? What if my water breaks at work? What if I cannot get hold of my husband?"

We could fill every day with the "what if" questions. We could stay awake nights imagining things that could go wrong. But what good does this do? One thing is for sure, we can easily feel paralyzed with fear when we obsess like this.

Dealing with facts in our lives can be much less stressful. Instead of thinking of the worst that could happen, we should say, "Stop!" and wait until we have more facts. The possibility of something going wrong exists, but statistics show the chance is low.

I ease my fears by remembering that most babies are born healthy.

Date / /

Today I Feel _____

Closeness

Day 225

During pregnancy, we may feel closer to our partner than ever before. We become more dependent for emotional support because this is the one person who has as much love for the baby as we do. Even though one person carries the baby, both experience the emotional ties.

Other times we may be concerned that the closeness seems absent. But those times may be when we're sorting things out on our own: our new roles as parents or the changes in our relationship. We need to trust that our Higher Power will guide each of us to our highest good as individuals, as a couple and as parents.

Part of being close to our partner is being open, especially when our life together is changing so rapidly.

Date / /

Today I Feel _____

Parenting Style

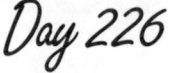

Day 226

As parents, we choose many different styles. Do we both believe in the same style? Is one of us flexible and the other more rigid? How do we function in situations when mutual support is crucial?

After the baby is born, we may not be cooperating with each other if we are operating in different directions. This will strain our marriage and also damage our relationship with our child. If we don't learn to compromise with each other, our children will grow up in a difficult situation. Now is the time to discuss our future parenting attitude and expectations before we find ourselves living it.

Even before birth, a discussion about childrearing is beneficial for me, my partner and certainly our child.

Date / /

Today I Feel

Childhood Pain

Day 227

Are we terrified of labor? Does this make us feel guilty or weak? We need to calm down and forgive ourselves. This reaction may be the result of early trauma in our lives, such as a car accident, surgery or illness. This memory may trigger anxiety about trusting our doctor or going to the hospital.

We need to learn how to relax. Our doctor can suggest methods, books and tapes. Some people find help in meditation, hypnosis or breathing techniques. If these methods don't help us, we might want to seek a therapist.

> *My childhood experiences will haunt me only if*
> *I let them. I fight back by learning to*
> *relax and letting go of the past.*

Date / /

Today I Feel _____

Feeling Good

Day 228

While we're pregnant, it's easy to let our appearance and conduct slip a little. As a result, our self-esteem and quality of life can slip, too. Why not use a little effort to retain a good feeling about ourselves?

Keeping up our appearance may lead us to supplement our tired old maternity wear. Perhaps we'd feel really good treating ourselves to a frilly maternity nightgown.

Our habits may need some brushing up, too, as we realize how much we bludgeon friends and family with endless pregnancy details.

I retain a good feeling now by taking care of myself in little ways.

Date / /

Today I Feel

Blended Family

Day 229

Our family may be considered a blended family because we have children from previous marriages. Even though we are very excited about having this first child together, the other family members may be feeling tense and unsure. At a time when we may be bursting with happiness, our home may be filled with anxiety and stress. As much as we want our stepchildren to rejoice in this new beginning and take part, we must understand that they may need the time and the space to accept this change gradually.

Patience, love and tender understanding are the ingredients needed for me to help my stepchildren through the transition of accepting the idea of a new member into our blended family.

Date / /

Today I Feel _____

_____

_____

_____

Coach

Day 230

To think we can make it through labor simply by reading, taking a Lamaze class and talking to friends is pretty courageous. There is one more important ingredient: the coach. Most women find labor much tougher than expected. Having someone there to talk us through contractions, bring us ice chips and massage our lower back helps us get through this experience.

The more our coach knows about labor, the more confident he or she will feel and the more useful they can be. A sensitive coach will not be absorbed in the pain and will have the mental strength to guide us well.

> *Just knowing I will not have to experience labor alone is already comforting.*

Date / /

Today I Feel _____

Making Time

Day 231

There isn't enough time to accomplish everything. If we had more hours, we could set aside time for our own needs. If we do not have enough time now, how will we manage once the baby enters our world?

What we don't realize is that we have all the time we need, but the problem is how we manage it. A lot of low priority items creep in and make demands. The minutes add up and pretty soon night falls and we haven't done what we intended.

The answer lies in our power to make the time for ourselves and our baby. By focusing on making the time now, we will be more prepared for the homecoming event.

***What I value receives top attention
and much dedicated effort.***

Date   /   /

Today I Feel

Procrastination

Day 232

All these projects have to get done before the baby arrives, right? Clothes, bedding, decorating, food. But with all this to do, why do we lounge on the sofa night after night?

Unfortunately, procrastination is an expectant mother's best friend. We think we have tons of time, but in reality forty weeks fly by. First, we need to admit we are procrastinating and then question the importance of all our plans. What tasks are really necessary? Next, perhaps we can ask our husband or a friend to help. When the inner leading gets strong enough, we'll find ourselves active again.

With the help of my friends, spouse and Higher Power, I trust that what's important will get done.

Date / /

Today I Feel

Ideals

Day 233

"I will never discuss my pregnancy with co-workers! I will never wear tennis shoes with a maternity dress! And I will certainly never bore everyone with ultrasound pictures!"

We may have made statements like this earlier in our lives. We listened with dismay as pregnant co-workers bored everyone and couldn't believe our girlfriend actually showed off her ultrasound photos. We would never sacrifice fashion for comfort like our neighbor waddling down the sidewalk in her tennis shoes. After all, when we got pregnant, we'd be in complete control with perfect style. Why is it then, that we find ourselves doing all of the above?!

In these days of real life pregnancy, I am gentle, forgiving and lighthearted with myself.

Date / /

Today I Feel _____

_____

_____

_____

Sex

Day 234

Sex at this point may be uncomfortable or even nonexistent. Our stomach is large and cumbersome, our bodies feel awkward and we are probably concentrating on everything but sex. We simply may not have the energy or interest.

This closeness can be replaced with other satisfying experiences. The emotional bonds can become closer now as we get ready to be parents.

Our love can be expressed verbally or with cuddling, kissing, hand holding and massage, or so-called "outercourse." Better verbal communication will help our relationship evolve into a deep friendship.

This phase of our lives together is only temporary, but it helps our love grow.

Date / /

Today I Feel _____

Prayer Power

Day 235

Silently emptying our minds, pouring out tears of concern and expressing thanks for the love around us are all ways of praying. This can take place whether we are in our beds talking to ourselves, whispering to the teddy bear in our infant's crib or kneeling in a church. Prayer provides strength, a mysterious source of energy and hope within us. Prayer provides direction and guidance in times of turmoil. It also provides us with a calm sense of inner peace.

Prayer does not have to be a recited piece we learned in church. It is a simple, sincere dialogue with our most trusted, loving friend. Prayer lifts us up beyond ourselves into a world that will show us the way.

My pregnancy becomes much more peaceful when I take time to pray.

Date / /

Today I Feel

Limits

Day 236

Are we feeling overwhelmed? Are we trying to do too much? Raising our children, being a companionable wife, going to night school, working? A good indication of being "overbooked" is when we stop enjoying what we used to love. The only solution is to set some limits.

Our number one priority now is a healthy pregnancy. Once the baby comes, that will change. But for now, anything that detracts from this goal needs to be set off to the side. This could mean taking the kids to our mother's so we can get a good night's sleep or saying no to being homeroom mother. We need to do what it takes to keep our priorities straight.

I set limits on what I take on and learn to say no to new responsibilities.

Date / /

Today I Feel _____

Sensations

Day 237

Many times we read that our baby can sense outside stimuli while still inside the womb. This information is an opportunity for us to introduce our baby to our home early. Let us take some time every day to treat our baby to some socialization.

While lying in bed next to us, Dad can accustom the baby to his voice and touch. The baby will notice the difference from our softer sounds and touches. Constant exposure to the dog's barking will prepare the baby for our home. Listening to our favorite music will also produce feelings of comfort and peace.

Our baby's world is enhanced even before birth when I take the time to introduce our household.

Date / /

Today I Feel

Focus

Day 238

To remain focused demands concentration, practice and discipline. In labor, we can either flounder around or we can choose to remain focused and in control as much as possible. Right now, we can't predict how intense labor will be, but by practicing our focus techniques, we will be better prepared.

We can begin by staring at one thing for periods of thirty seconds and build up to two minutes. While focusing on that one thing — a curtain rod, tennis shoe or crack in the wall — we need to totally block out everything around us. This experience is similar to being in a meditative state.

Help me, Greater Power, to have the discipline to practice focusing a little each day.

Date / /

Today I Feel

Strength

Day 239

Spiritually strong people may be intimidating to us. We wonder if their strength comes from having survived some suffering. We worry that we can't be spiritually strong because we haven't experienced suffering during our pregnancy or earlier in our lives.

We need to realize that through our Higher Power we can use our lives to help others and thereby strengthen ourselves spiritually. While pregnant, we can reach out to other pregnant women, listening and sharing information.

We can help others become knowledgeable, responsible and develop as human beings. Thus we ourselves become strong.

Let me do as I believe.
Let me develop spiritually.

Date / /

Today I Feel _____

Perfect Parents

Day 240

There is no such person as a perfect parent or perfect baby, since we all have limitations, weaknesses and fears. Perfectionism is something to strive for; to expect it from ourselves or our baby is only a setup for disappointment.

We have a vision of how we would like to see things and take steps to meet that goal. In the process we will become more familiar with our limitations. Part of striving for perfection is learning about our boundaries. The more we do this for ourselves, the easier it is to accept those we love.

*I work at accepting myself and my unborn child,
by letting go of my idea of perfect and accepting God's.*

Date / /

Today I Feel _____

A Gift

Day 241

One young man wanted nothing more than to be a father, but his wife had several miscarriages. Recently, they were both ecstatic when she was pregnant with twins. Unfortunately, she went into premature labor and lost the two girls. Months later, tears still come to his eyes as he tells about this experience.

We have all heard stories like this over the years. Some couples try to have children, yet for some reason cannot. This is when we wrap our arms around our swelling abdomen and tell ourselves how fortunate and grateful we are. We won't feel totally secure until after the birth, but we're already past the time when most miscarriages occur. We are very lucky.

Gifts like this have to be appreciated.

Date / /

Today I Feel _____

Work

Day 242

Many expectant women have ambivalence about returning to work. Of course, economics may make the decision for some, but others may have a choice. The period after birth is very important and we may be thinking about this a lot.

For now, the most comforting thing we can do is line up good child care. We need to spend time researching a baby sitter, family day care or day-care center. What environment do we feel most comfortable with? Is there a neighbor available? Does a local church offer day care? Once we have decided, we know that no matter what care we have, we'll still worry some.

*Even though I may change my mind later,
I set up my return to work and become
more secure with arrangements.*

Date / /

Today I Feel _____

Values

Day 243

What we believe in, what we cherish and how we behave all represent our values. They protect us from making bad decisions or mistakes.

Most of our values were established while growing up. Before our baby is born, we need to take a values inventory. Do we want to pass these values on to our children?

We will show the value of our children by respecting them for their individuality. We value the medical care we are getting. We also value the closeness of our support people. All of our values create an attitude toward life that we need to be aware of.

Good values are important to maintain a healthy life for me and my baby.

Date / /

Today I Feel _____

Prayer

Day 244

Let us pray that in the first hours of our baby's life he feels our warmth and companionship in his heart, soul and mind. We ask that God lead him into this life with the gift of faith and the strength to overcome fear. May our child be wrapped in the arms of loving grace and find peace and joy in our world.

Our child will be bound in body to the world and its earthly things, but also bound in spirit to God. May our baby find the love he will need along the road of life. May our baby grow and create a heart of joy, finding strength in God during times of difficulty.

God already has an infinite love for our child which will protect him all his life.

Date / /

Today I Feel

Sleep

Day 245

As well as invading our waking lives, this pregnancy is now affecting our sleep habits. We know we are supposed to sleep on our sides and some have said on the left side for the oxygen flow. But this can become difficult, especially if we are normally back or stomach sleepers.

In addition to position discomfort, we may be waking up every two hours to go to the bathroom or turn over (a major endeavor). We also are awakened by concerns about the baby. Whatever the reasons, our sleeping habits are seriously disturbed, which probably increases irritability.

I turn this negative into a positive as I see how nature is preparing me for the wake-up calls of a new baby.

Date / /

Today I Feel

New Habits

Day 246

For many days, months or years, we have conducted our lives in a certain manner. We have our routines that we follow from showering in the morning to watching the eleven o'clock news at night. Once our baby arrives, though, these routines will change.

Maybe it is time we take a look at some of the ways we spend our time. If we've been getting in a rut lately, we need to regain a little flexibility about life. Not to worry . . . adding a child to our household will tip all routines upside down! Older parents will especially appreciate this chance to escape boredom.

I stay open to go with the flow of the different routines of our new family member.

Date / /

Today I Feel

Temporary Condition

Day 247

We need to keep in mind that our present state is only temporary. We will not always be this heavy, inactive, emotional, fatigued and anxious. The present is only a short period of our lives, although at this point it doesn't seem that way. We can find comfort in the longer view, envisioning where we are going.

Soon enough our lives will be completely different. To avoid feeling overwhelmed, we can use our energy to prepare for our future. We can't waste the present brooding. Instead, let us find the strength to enrich the texture of our present by not putting off preparations.

*By remaining positive in preparations,
I am able to look back on the good.*

Date   /   /

Today I Feel _____

Breastfeeding

Day 248

When we first learned we were pregnant, perhaps we didn't hesitate to say "no way" to what we saw as the restrictions of breastfeeding. Now after carrying this child for many months, we may feel differently. Breastfeeding is a way of continuing this deep bond with our baby.

We still have time to decide. Now we need to investigate breastfeeding. Our resources include friends, our doctor, the library and our local LaLeche League. We need to find out about common problems, breast preparation and time involved.

*Whether I decide to breastfeed or not, I know
I will be a caring mother and my baby
will be healthy either way.*

Date / /

Today I Feel _____

_____

_____

_____

Relief

Day 249

Parental responsibility is a never-ending job. The transition to parenthood may not be as smooth as we anticipate. We will have many emotional reactions. At first we welcome the newness, but gradually our excitement becomes resentment and irritability.

Relief is the name of the game. Right now we need to line up people who can help us during the first weeks of parenthood. Aunts, mothers, neighbors and friends can all become part of our relief network. They can provide an important service that will help us keep our sanity.

I seek out a relief network to help me cope with the first weeks of constant baby duties and give me and my partner some time alone.

Date / /

Today I Feel _____

_____

_____

_____

The Baby's Sex

Day 250

"You're carrying so low, it must be a girl." "You're overdue, it must be a stubborn boy." "I had a dream you had twins!"

These are comments we hear often during our pregnancy. The predictions people make are astounding. But why not predict? After all, they have a fifty percent chance of being correct!

How valuable are these predictions? Probably not very. If we want to know the sex, we can find out during an ultrasound. The urge for people to predict and give advice comes from their need to participate in the event.

When people's comments drive me crazy, I smile and thank them for sharing with me.

Date / /

Today I Feel _____

Home

Day 251

Soon our home will be complete and our family together as one, caring for each other through the years ahead. Our home is where we build our lives through growth and change. Whether we realize it or not, we have grown tremendously during these last months. Our home has provided us with the support to endure the daily problems. In the near future, this will be the stabilizing force behind our baby's developing years. We will give our baby strength to face the ever-changing world. Home is our rock and fortress. Home is the place soon to be shared with our newborn and where we experience life's most beautiful relationships.

With God's help, I make our home a place of love and a blessing to all.

Date / /

Today I Feel _____

_____

_____

_____

Surrender

Day 252

The idea of detaching ourselves from others in our lives can be difficult. After all, don't we know best? Don't we know what needs to happen? The answer is sometimes, but not all the time.

People in our lives own their feelings and circumstances. It is not in our power to control them. The sooner we realize this, the better off we will be, especially as we prepare to be mothers.

There's no way to control a baby's rhythms, schedules and temperament. If we expect to control them, we will be in for a surprise.

I have greater peacefulness in parenting if I admit how powerless I am over my baby's routines.

Date / /

Today I Feel _____

Family Leave

Day 253

A sister may be talking about taking a leave from work or school to help us when the baby comes. In-laws may be planning to come in from out of town. Neighbors may say they'll stop in every day to check on us.

As much as we appreciate all the offers of help, we must remember that we'll be overwhelmed with the newness, possibly exhausted and looking forward to some quiet time in our own bed.

How do we envision our first hours at home? Do we want lots of help? Or do we want some time to get acquainted with the baby?

I think through what I'm going to need and communicate with those around me. There's a place for help!

Date / /

Today I Feel _____

Vision

Day 254

So much change is before us: our current lifestyle, our role as wife, our partner's role, our daily routines and responsibilities. One way to greet these changes is by creating a positive vision of our future. We start by seeing in our minds a fun, loving home shared with our baby. We can discuss with our husband, our other children and our parents how we plan to raise the baby. By focusing positively on our future, it will not seem as scary. As we look forward to this new person in our lives, we need to actively prepare ourselves and our family.

Having a positive vision grants me a sense of control and instills personal power.

Date / /

Today I Feel _____

Success

Day 255

How we define success during our pregnancy makes a big difference in how successful we feel about it. Some of us may say success is having a healthy baby without any problems during labor. Others will define it as not having a C-section, not using drugs and a labor less than three hours. Why do we define success as a definite outcome? Success can be measured daily before and after the actual birthing event occurs. Success can be defined as every time we reach for an apple instead of a candy bar. It means finding the personal strength not to drink coffee or smoke. Success is exercising positive thinking.

I refrain from setting expectations and see success in each day.

Date / /

Today I Feel

Twins

Day 256

If we find out we're carrying twins, we may find ourselves in a state of shock. Even though we may have done a good job of planning this pregnancy, we are caught by surprise by this one.

"This can't be happening! Why me? How will we ever manage?" We feel we'll have double the responsibilities of being a parent, and now have more doubts and anxieties. Why not take this energy and turn it into positive thinking?

Family and friends will probably spoil us and the babies twice as much. And most importantly, we will experience a good lesson in realizing what little control we have at times, a lesson that prepares us for the trials and tribulations of parenting.

Time will help me adjust and accept the reality of my twins, a truly special gift.

Date / /

Today I Feel _____

Medical Leave

Day 257

Our pregnancy may not be progressing as smoothly as we hoped. Maybe our bodies are not as strong as we thought. Ligaments may be strained, our back stiff with unbearable pain or possibly we are extremely swollen with water weight. Because of our condition and the possibility of related risks, our doctor may recommend or insist upon a medical leave of absence from work. Our first reaction may be to reject this idea. If we stay home, will we go stir crazy?

*My baby and I deserve to be off our feet
and out of pain to ensure the best of health.
A medical leave gives us both time for
needed rest and nourishment.*

Date / /

Today I Feel _____

Ties

Day 258

The child we bear will forever have ties with us. It is an unexplainable phenomenon, but one understood among mothers. There will always be a connection between our child and us. We can call it a feeling or a sense rooted in the depth of our soul. It is felt each time we look into our baby's eyes, hold the delicate little hand and kiss their precious toes. Our ties to each other will bind us together for a lifetime. Since we have been pregnant, these ties have been forming. No matter what anxieties we have, that special bond is developing every day. When we see our infant's face, our purpose in life will be redefined.

I commit myself to the privilege of motherhood this day and for all our years together.

Date / /

Today I Feel _____

Belief

Day 259

Being surrounded by positive, upbeat people during pregnancy helps us through some tough days. When others believe in us, we tend to feel more confident in our ability to handle the challenges ahead. Unless we believe in ourselves and the goals we want to achieve, we will end up shortchanged. Only we can take the responsibility to accomplish what we want to, mentally, physically and emotionally. We must remember that the burning desire to achieve our goals can only come from us.

*The deeper my inner convictions,
the stronger I feel every day.*

Date / /

Today I Feel _____

_____

_____

_____

Miracle Assistant

Day 260

Toward the end of our forty weeks, we feel anxious, tired or even bored with our condition. We keep saying, "Anytime now," and yet the days keep going by. All we can think about is our tiny, little newborn.

We must trust that our Higher Power is in control of the process of birth. We can find comfort in knowing that all along we have been helping God with this creation. Now we can look forward to helping in the miracle of birth. We need not fret about each new day that falls upon us, but instead we can rejoice in the knowledge that we are working closely with God to bring a new person into the world.

This is a rare opportunity in my life, to assist God in a miracle. I treasure each day and do not wish away my time.

Date / /

Today I Feel

Estimated Time Of Arrival

Day 261

All of us have been given a due date, which we have circled on our calendars. This becomes the focal point of all our plans as well as those of other family members. But many babies come late, especially first timers. It might be better to think of this date as "estimated," give or take a week or so.

Our date could be off for many reasons which our doctor can discuss with us. Our baby will come when it is ready. At all times, our doctor will monitor our condition to ensure that the baby is thriving. In the meantime we might as well enjoy this brief pre-baby time.

*I remain calm as I await the birth of my child,
who will obviously live by its own schedule.*

Date   /   /

Today I Feel

Movement

Day 262

Our baby has been growing so quickly the last eight months. We have enjoyed a lot of movements and kicking! Now that delivery is almost here, the baby is bigger and more cramped. There is less room to move around and less movement.

We may feel alarmed at first and then perhaps a little lonely. Although we realize this is preparation for birth, we may still feel concern. We need to discuss this with our physician to relieve our anxiety. We are even more comforted when we turn these concerns over to our Higher Power.

In addition to the knowledge I obtain from my doctor, I relieve worry by giving cares over to my Higher Power.

Date / /

Today I Feel

Stages

Day 263

During the first trimester, we had the following symptoms: fatigue, nausea and increased urination. During the second, our pregnancy became more real as we "popped out." That's when we thought we looked so cute in maternity clothes. Somewhere along the line we began the third or "waddle" stage. This soon will develop into the "drop" stage, as the baby descends into birth position. For most, this is the final stage, but for some, there is the "shuffle" yet to go. This is not defined in any books, but we know when it is happening. We develop hip, lower back or leg pressures and problems due to the weight of the dropped baby. Truly, this had better be the final stage! It is mentally relieving for me to joke about my ailment.

Humor helps me practice for parenting.

Date / /

Today I Feel

Uncertainty

Day 264

"How will I know when real labor begins?" "When should I call the doctor?" "When do I go to the hospital?" All these questions race through our minds. Even if we have gone to Lamaze classes and read all the books, we still wonder, "How will I know?"

The classes or reading may not be too reassuring about this part of our pregnancy. What can be comforting is knowing that our medical advisors are there for us, morning, noon or night. That's their job. When we are in doubt about whether we are experiencing real labor, we can call and be soothed by an expert opinion.

I may misjudge the onset of labor, but I know that it's better to call and find out than not to call and put my baby at risk.

Date / /

Today I Feel _____

Moving On

Day 265

Not wanting something to end is a bittersweet emotion. Before starting our journey through pregnancy, we were different in so many ways. We were filled with wonder about pregnancy and awe as it developed. We were lovers with our husbands, not the close friends we are now. We had a whole new experience ahead, not knowing the depth at which it would change us.

Instead of viewing birth as an end, we should think of it as the beginning of something that will last much longer than nine months. May we acknowledge the beauty of our nine months, let it go and embrace the future.

*I ride the wave of peaceful fulfillment from
my pregnancy as I reach motherhood.*

Date / /

Today I Feel _____

Waiting

Day 266

The final weeks of pregnancy are here. At times it probably seemed as if it would never arrive. Other times, it felt as if time was passing way too swiftly. Now that the end is in sight, we start to play the "waiting game." Patience is the key to enjoying our final weeks. Our baby will come when it's ready. We can be sure of that. Our individual needs, wants or requests may not be met. All we can do is take one day at a time, remain calm and try to enjoy these last days. We have put in a lot of hard work, so let's just sit back in peace and confidence knowing we have done everything in our power to get to this point.

I savor these remaining days and remind myself that this is not a race.

Date / /

Today I Feel _____

Nesting

Day 267

The windows in our home have been thoroughly washed and the sills scrubbed down. The closets and junk drawers are organized for the first time in years. The cupboards are full of enough food to last for months. What is happening? We envisioned spending the last weeks peacefully awaiting labor. Instead, we are attacking household chores and even reorganizing the Christmas card list. We are experiencing pre-labor nesting. Just as birds spend days preparing their homes for the spring brood, our body feels more energetic prior to birth. We need to be sure not to overextend ourselves and save energy for labor.

Nothing is wrong with housecleaning, but I follow my inner leading and don't overexert.

Date / /

Today I Feel _____

Medication

Day 268

Before we decide on medication during labor, we need to know what is available, pros and cons, and when it can be administered. Having a thorough understanding will prepare us for possible changes during the actual event.

We may be against the use of drugs because it's better for the baby, but if we are stuck at a certain stage, our doctor may recommend medication.

On the other hand, we may feel we have no threshold for pain and want to be "knocked out" from the beginning. By discussing these concerns with our doctor, friend and spouse, we learn about all the options to help us through birth.

I am open to whatever comes; no one can predict completely how labor will go.

Date / /

Today I Feel _____

Prelabor Signs

Day 269

We feel in tune with our bodies, awaiting signs of labor. Every little pain, sharp cramp or mounting pressure makes us ask, "Is this it?"

We need once again to remind ourselves of the difference between prelabor and real labor. Our due date is approaching and we need to be prepared. Prelabor signs help us learn how to react and give us an idea of what real labor will be like. How do we react to false labor? Frightened? Elated? Emotional? Now is a good time to get our minds ready for what is to come.

I become discouraged when I continue to experience prelabor, but I know this builds confidence for the real thing.

Date / /

Today I Feel _____

Big Picture

Day 270

Looking at the big picture helps us put things in the right perspective, particularly when we feel trapped. We do not have the baby yet, and this may cause some negative feelings. We feel we have waited long enough and deserve to have birth behind us. If we continue to dwell on these thoughts, we will continue to feel down.

We can safely say that one month from now we will be home holding our baby in our arms. We can honestly say that we are at the end of our pregnancy. Approximately one year from now, we will be celebrating our child's first birthday.

By looking at the big picture, I find peace, even at this stage of pregnancy.

Date / /

Today I Feel _____

Overdue Addendum

Overdue

Day 271

For nine months we have had a magical due date implanted in our minds. Numerous plans have been made around it: the baby's room, maternity leave, family members' vacations and prenatal classes. The due date comes, and then it passes by.

We are now in the "overdue" category. This is a time when we are bombarded with phone calls from neighbors, work, family and friends. We wake up in the morning saying, "Today could be the day." This is when patience is sorely tested.

Do we consider ourselves patient? Is our partner patient? If we don't know, we'll find out during this waiting time. And once again, it's good learning for motherhood!

Patience is allowing life to unfold before me, in peace and serenity. Patience is healthy.

Date / /

Today I Feel

Inducing

Day 272

We have so looked forward to signs of labor when we can tell our partner we had better go to the hospital. However, now we are overdue and our doctor is recommending we go into the hospital to be induced. Somehow it seems as if we're being robbed of the mystery of labor happening naturally. We had such high expectations! However, this is a time when we have to become "bottom-line" thinkers: labor is labor, no matter how it comes on. Our focus needs to remain on our health and delivering a healthy baby. This is also a good time to talk with our Higher Power and friends who have gone through this.

Being induced doesn't have to be a problem if I create a mindset that focuses on a healthy baby waiting to be born.

Date / /

Today I Feel _____

_____

_____

_____

Advice

Day 273

"Drive down a bumpy road!" "Have sex every day!" "Scrub the kitchen floor!" "Go walk the mall and shop till you drop!" "Take a long, hot shower!" "Drink a couple of glasses of wine!"

Do any of these sound familiar? Again, we are the recipient of unneeded advice. People seem to think the above suggestions will bring on labor, but in fact, after all that, we'd be too tired to greet it properly!

Our doctor is monitoring us to ensure all is well. People mean well and are only excited about the pending birth. Our baby will come when it's the right time. The apple will fall from the tree when it is ready.

I will smile nicely, ignore them all and consult my doctor if it becomes necessary.

Date / /

Today I Feel _____

Final Preparations

Day 274

Mounting excitement is what we feel at times throughout our overdue weeks. We made it so far and now, the real waiting begins. If we hate to wait for anything, this can be a challenging time.

The first rule is to keep busy so the time will seem to go by faster. We can enjoy these unstructured days for special projects or time with the family. Each day we can make a realistic to-do list, so we keep busy but don't overdo.

The second rule is to stay relaxed. Through meditation or quiet time, we stay in touch with our emotions and our Higher Power. The last rule is remembering that eventually birth will occur.

*I arrange my time to relax but keep busy
in preparation for the arrival.*

Date / /

Today I Feel

Special Attention

Day 275

Being past due, we now have to see our doctor more frequently and may have extra medical tests. These are routine steps to ensure the health of mother and baby. At first, we may be anxious, but we can learn from this and find comfort. We can take the opportunity to find out more about the procedures for testing, labor, delivery and recovery. We can discuss the experience with our doctor or with friends. This will provide additional support during a time when we may be feeling a little discouraged and frustrated.

I put my emotions aside and learn from these experiences to be even more prepared for the birthing process.

Date / /

Today I Feel _____

Ebbing Energy

Day 276

As we reheat spaghetti, we realize this is the third day in a row we've had frozen dinners or leftovers in front of the TV. What is happening to us? Where are the days of homemade meals and dinner together? Our normal routine is nonexistent and we've become sluggish and unmotivated.

We're experiencing a kind of grieving, reconciling ourselves to being overdue. Our expectations are not being met.

This is part of the ebb and flow of being overdue. We need to turn it around by refocusing our energies or we will be forced to do so by the onset of labor, which will happen at some point!

I may not feel very energetic right now. I just want to "exist," but this is okay — it's not forever.

Date / /

Today I Feel _____

Emotional Balance

Day 277

Is this wait starting to make us nervous? Are we beginning to hoard anger inside of us or take it out on others?

Our emotions can be very powerful. We put up our defensive shell and sometimes don't let anyone peel it away. We find ourselves ticked off at everyone and flying off the handle easily. Communicating our feelings to those close to us will help keep us on balance.

Just as important is taking the time to find out what is going on inside of us. Is our anger masking other emotions like fear or worry?

I turn to a sympathetic ear to help me sort out these powerful emotions. I also spend time with myself and my Higher Power.

Date / /

Today I Feel _____

The Blahs

Day 278

We've done a good job keeping busy these last few weeks, but being overdue makes us slump and perhaps develop a case of the "blahs." The only thing we think will rescue us will be the birth of our child.

All the excitement about the due date is subsiding. We may feel as if we have lost control over our lives. After all, quitting or just plunging ahead is not possible.

We need a quick fix. Take a break! Ask a family member to come along and get out of the house. Go to a museum, have lunch out or take a walk in the park. The main point is to get out of ourselves and into the world with others.

I take action today to clear my head of the "blahs" and get out of my rut.

Date / /

Today I Feel _____

Euphoria

Day 279

No makeup ... wild hair ... an old bathrobe ... frequent eating, trips to the bathroom. This may describe our life as we wait to go into labor. We seem to "just exist" until awakened by a phone call from our husband saying there's a party at his brother's house. Some event presents itself and we muster enough energy to get out of our hibernating cycle and back into the swing of life.

Surprisingly, we may feel euphoric while away from the house. The stimulation of being around other people living normal lives is excellent for our morale. Our energy returns and we come home with a lighter heart.

*Soon I'll be able to live a normal,
more enriched life again.*

Date / /

Today I Feel _____

Closing Prayer

Day 280

Today we may not know what to think. We're so tired, physically and emotionally. When we feel like this, a special meditation or prayer can help.

Holy Spirit, what I ask this evening is guidance and strength for the time ahead.
Stay near and keep me from fear.
Help me to know I can depend on those around me. Give support to my medical team and family. Help me fulfill this dream joyfully. Into your care I give my life, my future and my unborn child.

I take comfort in simple meditations or prayers before
I lie down to rest, leaving my mind empty and far from effort.

Date / /

Today I Feel _____

Strength

Day 281

Our pregnancy trip has somehow become bumpy and slow, whereas at one time it was smooth and quick. We started off with a full tank of gas in a race car, but now we are running on fumes with a draining battery. We used to enjoy our days and filled them with sleepy dreams of our baby. But now, everything is tedious and tiring.

This is, however, a small price to pay for the precious gift we will be receiving. We are in a transition period that will soon be over. What strength we may be lacking physically we can make up for spiritually. Thinking positively, envisioning our future, and recalling pleasant memories can strengthen our spirit.

I need to remember that all my vitality will be renewed in good time.

Date / /

Today I Feel

Welcome Home

Day 282

There is a light at the end of the tunnel. That day comes when we take our beautiful precious baby home. No woman is pregnant forever. Although things may not go as we imagined, we will bring our baby home very soon.

We must remember the ebb and flow of life. All the difficult moments we experienced while we waited are replaced in an instant as we look into our baby's eyes for the first time. All the confusion dissolves as our fingers are grasped by that little hand. All the worries vanish when we gaze at the angelic infant peacefully sleeping in our arms.

I am caught in a difficult transition period,
but I have confidence that many beautiful
moments are yet to come.

Date / /

Today I Feel

Changes

Day 283

On the shelf above the fireplace, someday soon, there will be a picture of our beautiful baby and maybe even a family portrait. There will also be a photo from the hospital of our newborn on the first day of life. All of this proof of change will surround us. We may wonder how this can be when the house is so still and quiet now. As we sit and ponder over this impending change, the powerfulness of its reality can be shocking. One day our life is one way, and the next day, BOOM, it's completely different. It will be totally changed, never to return to the present state. A new sense of normal will be created and before we know it, we will feel as if we have always known our baby. We will not even be able to imagine life without children.

God, hold our family in the light of love.

Date / /

Today I Feel _____

_____

_____

_____